I0439975

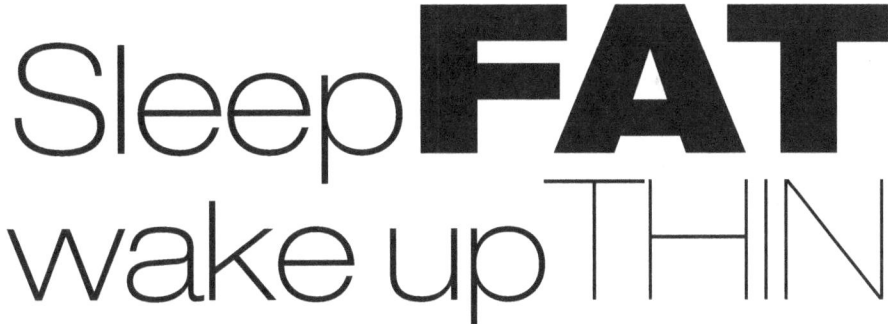

Sleep **FAT**
wake up THIN

How To Lose Weight **F.A.S.T** Without Struggle

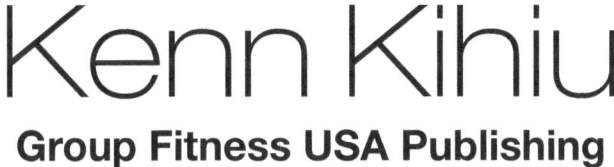

Kenn Kihiu

Group Fitness USA Publishing

Sleep Fat Wake Up Thin
How To Lose Weight F.A.S.T Without Struggle

By Kenn Kihiu

Copyright © 2013 by Kenn Kihiu for Group Fitness USA Publishing

ISBN: 1481948067
ISBN-13: 9781481948067

First edition published 2013

Disclaimer

The techniques, ideas and suggestion in this document are not intended as a substitute for proper medical advice. Always consult your physician or health care professional before performing any new exercise, exercise technique or before starting a new diet program. – Particularly if you are pregnant, nursing, elderly or if you have any chronic or recurring conditions. Any application of the techniques, ideas and suggestions in this document is at the reader's sole discretion and risk.

The authors of this document make no guarantees or warranties of any kind in regard to the content of this document, including but not limited to, any implied warranties or merchantability or fitness for any particular purpose. The authors shall not be held liable or responsible for any misunderstanding or misuse of the information contained in this manual or for any loss, damage, or injury caused or alleged to be caused directly or indirectly by any treatment, action, or application of any food or food source discussed in this manual. The authors of this document are not liable or responsible to any person or entity for any errors contained in this document, or if any special incidental, or consequential damaged caused or alleged to be caused directly or indirectly by the information contained within. The statements in this book have not been evaluated by the U.S. Food and Drug Administration. This information is not intended to diagnose, treat, cure, or prevent any disease

Table of Contents

MODULE 3

- The Basics Of your Body's Acid & Alkaline Balance
- How to easily Alkalize your body
- What To Eat In Abundance
- What Good Fats to consume
- Water – Essence of Life and eating your water

MODULE 4

- How weight loss really happens
- Uncover the lies about frequency of food
- Short and Flexible Fasting Defined
- Dispelling The Misinformation
- Breakfast is necessarily not the most important meal of the day

MODULE 5

- The ABC's of Weight Loss
- Getting Your Mind and Body In Sync
- Mental Tools For Handling Emotional Eating
- How To Help Your Body Control Appetite and Cravings

- What Exactly Should You Eat?
- "Real Food" Guidelines
- Making Comfort Food More Comforting

- Life is more fulfilling when we pay it forward

The End...

YES! You are in the right place because this is where it all *starts!* However let me give away the ending to this course and the journey you are about to take. You will become truly aware of the power you have over your life and your health. You finally will have the right tools and knowledge and for once and for all, lose the extra weight you carry and maintain a healthy lifestyle.

You will be totally free. Free from the control food has over your life. You will be free to enjoy your life and even on occasion, eat foods you thought were forbidden and still enjoy them without gaining a single pound.

You will be filled with the kind of confidence you get when you know your body is life's greatest gift. You will be an inspiration to your family and friends and you will make a difference to the lives of those you love with the energy and vitality only a healthy body can bring.

This course will be life transforming and I cannot wait to hear your success story. In our time together, you will learn not only how to lose the weight you've always wanted to lose but also how to get healthy and have more energy than you thought you could ever have.

The Journey

Now I may not know you personally, but it is safe to say that I know something about you. Just by buying this course – you've shared that you're ready to take your health seriously. You're ready to change.

After you've been around the block a few times you come to realize that the body is life's greatest gift. At least, that's what I believe. The body is the instrument we use to make our hopes and dreams come true and my wish for you is an extraordinary life; one filled with health, happiness and success.

One of the factors that determine our success is how well we can deliver on our promises. You've invested in this course and I want you to make the promise that you will go through this whole course and complete it. Most people who buy this course will never even remove the shrink wrap. You're already doing great!

You are different, so let's keep up that motivation and energy. Go through each module, remembering it's not a race if it takes you a few weeks, that's okay. The goal is to finish what you've started and to let the knowledge and information I will share with you, sink into and work in your life.

I also want you to know that are not alone in this journey because you have a true partner in me. I'm going to help you by making this material easy to consume. I don't want to bore you with the things I know about biochemistry. It really doesn't matter in the long run about the 'why,' but it matters more that you learn what works for long term healthy weight loss. With a minimum of scientific jargon, I will show you the blueprint, the map to how you will achieve your weight loss goal.

So what results can you expect? Well it depends on the person, but I promise you this, you will get to your weight loss goal even if you put half of what we talk about it into practice. Let me ask you, how many pounds do you need to shed before you reach your ideal, healthy weight?

10? 30? 100?

Whatever your answer, multiply it by 3.

You are now looking at the number of days it will take for you to reach your ideal weight when you follow my program. For those with a lot of weight to lose it will happen even faster.

All this, without constantly feeling deprived plus gaining a lot of energy and vitality.

You will have also a lot of **a-ha** moments along the way, even without Oprah. You will notice that old struggles aren't so hard. Because you will find out the secret that no one else knows: hormones are to blame for your weight gain.

Think about it: A woman who is pregnant will gain weight regardless of how little food she eats. With all of those hormones surging through her body, they're telling her that she needs to gain weight. And she does.

Hormones are chemicals released by your cells or glands that send out a message that will affect other cells or glands in the body. If you can change the hormone levels in your body, you can change your metabolism. And it doesn't take much work – just a few simple changes to your diet. Yes, really.

Your body is nature's perfect pharmacy and it will produce the right hormones, in the right quantities and deliver it to the right target organ without side effects and all you have to do is make better dietary choices. Your body is ready to change the way it behaves at the drop of a dime, but you need to learn how to make the best choices for the weight loss you want.

By the way, I'm not a purist. I believe moderation is the key to life. I want this to be a lifestyle and it should not be about depriving yourself so you will not find a lot of restrictions with my plan. I'm not going to tell you to eat nothing but kale or to suck on an ice cube when you're hungry.

If you can't maintain this plan, then what's the point?

I confess I am not a dietician, nutritionist or someone trying to convince you to go on a fad diet. Instead what I will do is provide you with simple recommendations. Try some, try them all. It's up to you. You don't have to suffer through a small number of 'acceptable' recipes, complex point counting charts, or rules on the percentage of carbs, proteins, or fats to consume. My goal is to have you make small changes to your current diet, small changes that add up to big results.

This course will change your life. It really will. For some of you, the title will prove true, one day after following my system and adopting some of the principles, you'll wake up, put on those pants or step on the scale and say, "Wow that was easy. It really felt like I went to sleep fat and woke up thin." Heck, you might even get up before your alarm to enjoy that feeling.

Tales of Deception

Food is a controlled substance. Stay with me here. Just like alcohol and tobacco, there are rules that govern the manufacture, importation, possession, use, and distribution of it. This means if you follow the money, you begin to see that the control is entirely in the hands of huge corporations that really determine what we eat. *(If you have a chance, please watch the movie "Food, Inc." You quickly get the idea of how powerful the food industry truly is.)*

The weight loss industry is a $60 billion industry – they want your money and need you to keep buying and purchasing their products. If you're healthy and thin, then they're not going to make money. Think about that for a minute. When you're sick and fat, you're a dollar sign and a new house and a new boat and their kid's college education.

Profit is their main goal and they want you to keep buying. These corporations invest heavily in lobbying and advertising. Not surprisingly, they spend more on marketing than on research and development. They are more interested in their bottom line rather than your waistline.

Scary? You decide. Many of the diseases we face today - obesity, type 2 diabetes, and high cholesterol - are not true diseases but symptoms of underlying conditions brought on by the things we eat. These conditions are easily fixable with changes in the simple choices that we make everyday without thinking. It's time to start thinking more.

Your miracle

I'm in love with the human body. What a gift you have, if you think about it. Your heart beats over 100,000 times a day. If all your muscles pulled in one direction, you would be able to pull a couple of Hummers. Did you know that size for size your tongue is the strongest muscle in your body? (No wonder we love to eat!) Your thigh bone, pound for pound, is stronger than steel? What truly happens inside your body is nothing short of miraculous and all you have to do is give it more of what it really needs.

If you follow my system, you will lose the weight, burn fat, gain energy, and feel healthy – the best you will have felt in years. Even though all of that sounds great, what you're really getting from this course is the chance to regain power and control over your own life.

Some of the things I'm going to share with you will sound crazy. I know it. I've heard it over and over again. But everything I recommend is backed by science but even more importantly, by a little common sense.

This course goes against what the current food and diet industry suggests. Let's just say I'm not expecting a Nobel Prize for this book or an interview with the Surgeon General.

But it works. I've seen it work. I've done the research. And you get to see the results.

How To Use This Course

This course is divided into 5 modules: One foundation module focuses on your mindset, which holds the secret ingredient to your success, and four nutrition modules which cover the acronym F.A.S.T.

F is for Fasting, Short and Flexible
A for Alkalinity and Water
S for Sugar and Insulin
T is for Taming Appetite, Behavior, and Cravings.

The objective with each module is
1.   Understand the module goal
2.   Understand the module principles. There is some scientific information here, but I have made it very easy to understand. Knowledge is at the foundation of motivation. For example, if you really like cooking and are good at it, chances are you want to learn new recipes and you are always eager to experiment with different foods. The more you know about something, the more motivation you have to do more with it.
3.   I will give you the how to's, the do's and don'ts and a summary of how to really make this plan your own.

This course will give you practical advice to turn yourself into a fat burning machine.

As a final word of preparation, let me offer a suggestion that will help you get this material and make it part of your life. This course was designed to build on itself. Begin with the first module first, then proceed with the second module second, the third module, third etc.

Many will start losing weight and be so successful with just one module that you might be tempted to forget the rest. If you do this, you're short-changing yourself. Go through this course from beginning to end.

You can't change your life if you don't get started. So are you ready?

MODULE 1

Your Philosophy – The Secret Sauce of Success

Your Mindset Determines Everything

The first module is the most important because it affects everything you do. I believe the mind is the key to everything. If you weigh more than you should, don't like to exercise, or cannot seem to keep yourself motivated, it's because of your life philosophy or mindset. While what you eat and how you move matter, if your mind isn't in the game, you're not going to eat well or move more.

You want to learn how to integrate your life and your pursuit of health so they complement each other without draining you of time, resources, or energy. To be successful with implementing any new changes in your life, you have to embrace some new life philosophies. Here are five important ones you should adopt in your life.

New Mindset #1:
Take 100% Responsibility For Your Life

Let me define philosophy as your personal beliefs about life and how you respond to life situations. Notice I said respond and not react. There is a difference between those two words. For example, you don't want to hear your doctor say that your body is reacting to the medication. You would rather hear you are **responding** well to the treatment.

Most people live a life where they react to situations instead of responding. You are driving down the highway and some person cuts right in front of you almost causing you a heart attack. You could react by taking it personally and as a result, get stressed, angry, increase your blood pressure, and think the world is out to get you. Or you could respond by not taking it personally and getting all tied up in knots about it and head on your merry way. We probably will never ever see that person again, so why ruin your day by being upset?

I want you to start thinking of the word responsibility as something you do rather than something you are. If you look closely at the word 'responsibility' it comes from two words 'respond' and 'ability'. Responsibility is the ability to choose your response and not just react to what life throws at you.

We are often not responsible for all the bad things that happen to us. However, we should claim responsibility when they do. Taking 100% responsibility for your life is taking ownership of everything that is happening or not happening in your life.

And this is not easy because we avoid responsibility at all costs. We complain, whine, make excuses, and blame our parents, spouses, friends, boss, economy, etc. Taking responsibility is not about assigning blame to you or to anyone else.

Far from it.

This is about saying, "I now own whatever is happening to me," even when it seems unfair. In fact especially when it seems unfair, you should be taking responsibility.

Give up all your victim stories and excuses. Give up blaming others for your lot in life. Give up complaining about what you are going through. If you avoid taking responsibility for you life, you welcome stress into your life; one of the biggest environmental cues for hunger and increased appetite.

Stress activates the body's response to threat or danger. It's called the fight, flight or freeze response. During this reaction, certain hormones like adrenaline and cortisol are released, increasing your heart rate and blood pressure, while slowing digestion and preventing you from burning fat.

Reacting to life gets you into trouble because it increases your stress levels. It puts your mind and body at a disadvantage. To be successful with your new goals in life, you must take 100% responsibility for your life. Nothing less will do.

New Mindset #2:
The Secret of The Easy Things

The easy things make all the difference. You will be successful if you constantly do the simple stuff. Buster Martin at the age of 102 in 2008 walked the entire London Marathon that is 26.2 miles in 10 hours. Think about that. He has never been a superstar athlete, but just a regular Joe who still goes to work every day. When he was asked what workout keeps him so fit, he said pushups. He does pushups every day. Think about that, something that is easy that anyone can do.

This is the secret of successful people; they seem to do the easy things every single day.

Some fruits and veggies with your meals – easy.

Weighing yourself regularly – easy.

Drink water often – easy.

But this is what trips people up because **if something is easy to do then it's easy <u>NOT</u> to do.**

Do you know that the biggest problem in medicine is? It's getting people to take their medicine. Sounds ridiculous, doesn't it? Even with the threat of death, people still don't take their medication. I know we have all done it, but, seriously, how easy is it to take 2 pills with a glass of water?

It's easy to do, but then again easy <u>not</u> to do.

If you consistently do the easy stuff I mention in this course, you will experience a breakthrough. Doing the easy stuff consistently means you start coming to terms with loving the process and not just the destination. And it's easy.

Consistently doing the easy stuff is the difference between those who succeed and those who fail.

New Mindset #3:
Happily Pay The Price in Advance

There is a Spanish proverb that says, "God says take all that you want but pay the price first." How often has this come true in your own life?

We live in a culture where people value the word FREE, where most people want something for nothing, but I'm sorry, you cannot reap if you don't sow and you cannot have a return on investment without the investment. In short, you can't get anything for free, even if it seems like you do at first.

Paying the price is saying in advance that you will do whatever it takes and you will find a way to make it happen. If you continue to stuff yourself with chocolate cake every day, you might have the satisfaction and the 'free' feeling of being happy. But down the road, you're going to pay the price. Jack LaLanne loved to say "A second on your lips and a lifetime on your hips !"

There is a price to pay for everything.

It's either the price of regret or the price of discipline. Be willing to pay the price of discipline and let me add <u>willingly</u> and <u>happily</u>. Don't complain or gripe, just do what needs to get done.

New Mindset #4:
Create Automatic Decisions

All change begins with a decision. So make your decision about what you want. I need to emphasize that this is about what <u>you</u> want because if you are doing this for others you will never truly be free.

Decide what you want and then decide in advance that you will stick to your decision, regardless of circumstances. Don't make your decisions dependent on variables such as weather or what your friends are thinking because you are setting yourself up for prompt failure.

Remember, it's not a decision unless it's completely independent of your circumstances; circumstances change all the time. If you decide that this is a good week to exercise then what happens next week, when it's not a good time anymore? Bye-bye decision.

Don't let circumstances change your ability to follow through on commitments.

Here is the trick; set up your life in such a way that you don't have to continuously make decisions about important things. You wake up in the morning and brush your teeth because it's an automatic decision you made many years ago and not one you have to decide on every day. You don't go to bed at night and wake up in the morning deciding whether you will brush your teeth. Well, hopefully not anyway.

I want you to set up many of the things we'll talk about in this course as automatic decisions so you can commit to them. Scientists have proven that willpower is a limited resource, meaning you can use it all up. So the more you use your willpower to make you do certain things, the less of it you have to accomplish the next round of tasks.

Set up your life so you don't have to make a decision. If tomorrow you have yet to decide whether you will exercise or not, then you will have to use your willpower to make that decision. You still have to decide what to wear, what exercises to do, how much weight to lift and before you know it you have used all your willpower and you haven't even begun exercising yet!

Learn to set up your life so you don't always have to make a decision.

New Mindset #5:
Think Of Progress Not Perfection

Face it, most people fail at reaching their goals because they want to be perfect. Stop it! Perfection is absolutely the worst standard you can set for yourself because it's impossible to achieve.

As human beings we seem to have a very short memory and we forget that we never succeeded at most of the things we did for the very first time. If you go through all the things you have accomplished, you will see that you stumbled in the beginning. We weren't perfect the first time we learned how to walk, ride a bike, or drive a car.

As a toddler did you say, "I quit trying to walk because every time I try to walk I keep falling on my butt"? Of course NOT! You kept on trying, slowly improving until one day it all clicked.

The **secret** to success is being **kind** and **gentle** to yourself. Stop beating yourself up and feeling guilty when you veer off course. Feeling guilty and beating yourself up for not being perfect is absolutely the worst way to make yourself a better person. You might move forward then backslide a bit, don't worry that's the way the process goes. Just don't wallow in guilt and beat yourself up.

The truth about guilt is that it often makes things worse. Feeling guilty over eating a chocolate cake will only make you eat more chocolate cake in the future. Step 1 is no guilt. Miss a workout? – don't beat yourself up. Have a bad eating day? - don't feel guilty.

I'm going to teach you something more powerful than guilt; and it's called awareness.

Enjoy what your eating even if it's bad for you, Instead of asking all those guilty questions like (Why can I never wake up and workout? Why can I never stop eating chocolate cake?), ask better questions like: <u>What</u> triggered the craving? Really what triggered this? And <u>What</u> are you going to do next time?

If you promise to workout in the mornings and you miss your workout, don't feel guilty and beat yourself up for not following through. Instead ask "<u>how</u> can I make it easier to workout in the mornings" or "<u>what</u> other times are better for me to exercise? Ask yourself <u>what</u> you can do to make it more convenient?

When you ask the "What and How" questions you begin to take 100% responsibility and start to solve the problem. Asking **what** and **how** is more powerful than just asking why, which looks to assign guilt and blame. Instead of blaming yourself or others, focus on taking action. Imperfect action Yes!; Because action is what starts to move you in the right direction.

Module 1: Summary

Adopt these new mindsets
- Take 100% responsibility for your life
- Learn & master the secret of doing the easy things

- Happily pay the price in advance
- Create automatic decisions
- Think of progress not perfection

If you do all five of these things most days, you are well on your way. But the least I can ask of you is to harness the power of doing the simple, easy things each and every day. They will make all the difference.

MODULE 2

Sugar and Fiber

The Sugar Problem

If you consume too much sugar, you will get fat. That is as simple as I can put it. But the problem we all face when it comes to sugar is there is a real reason why we like it and why the addiction is hard to break. It's like a torrid love affair, the more we have, the more we want and then it just consumes us and we get into a lot of trouble.

Almost all attempts to stop consuming sugar are truly difficult and usually end up in failure because, how do you stop consuming something that is generally widely accepted and something that you genuinely like and may even be addicted to?

The taste for sugar is a genetic weakness and this horrible love affair we have with sugar grows every year. Researchers believe that we eat up to 50 teaspoons of sugar that is about 200 grams of sugar every day! That is over 150 pounds of sugar a year. 200 years ago, that number was under 15 grams per day or about 12 pounds per year.

Our Pre-Historic Need For Sugar

Our bodies like the sweet taste of sugar and nature designed it that way. (So it's not really your fault.) Vitamins, minerals and fiber are not all that delicious by themselves so nature made fruits sweet so that we would eat those healthy apples, oranges, etc. Food manufacturers have exploited this sweet fact and the emergence of refined sugar has contributed to fat gains.

Refined sugar is called a drug by some because during the refining process everything of food value is removed and what is left has a direct chemical effect on the body. If you are not sure sugar is a drug, then give kids some candy and you will see insanity prevail right in front of your eyes.

One of the biggest problems we face is that most folks at one time or another realize that they have to stop eating too much sugar. What does not work is just removing the sugar from your diet without eliminating the underlying reason why your body is craving it.

It's Not Just In The Mind

Sugar craving is not just in your mind or a psychological thing. There are chemicals and physiological reasons for it and scientists are now beginning to understand how eating sugar affects our "feel-good" neurotransmitters such as serotonin. Also, there are many other physical causes for sugar cravings: acidity, overgrown yeast in the blood, and stress.

How Sugar Makes You Fat - Understanding The Basics of Insulin

The hormone insulin is completely essential to life. In the right amounts, your body functions like a well-oiled machine, but in excess you begin storing fat - especially around your belly. Bottom line, if you have too much body fat, you probably have too much insulin floating around in your body. It's the reason insulin is known as the fat storing hormone, because if you chronically have increased levels of insulin, you will become fat and stay fat.

Every time you eat, the food is broken down into glucose, the simplest sugar that the body's cells use for energy. A rise in your blood sugar causes the release of the hormone Insulin by the pancreas. So if you want to lose fat and keep it off, you have to understand how this very important hormone works.

Adults have about 5 liters of blood being pumped through the body. To give you an idea 5 liters is about 14 cans of coke. Now think about this, for just those 5 liters of blood, you need only about one teaspoon of sugar for basic functioning.

The more sugar you have in your blood, the thicker it becomes. (Think maple syrup or honey.) Your body wants to continue circulating the blood so you can live, so when you have more than a teaspoon of sugar in your bloodstream and your body is not burning it, insulin is secreted by the pancreas. This process instructs the liver and muscles to take the blood sugar and store it in your muscles and liver as glycogen.

But wait, there is more. You have limited reserves of glycogen and if your liver and muscles cannot store more of the sugar as glycogen then the **excess sugar is converted to fat tissue very rapidly.**

To make matters worse, when your insulin levels are high, the use of fat as an energy source comes to a complete stop.

If You Keep Shouting I'll Stop Listening

If you continue consuming lots of sugary foods, your cells become bombarded with insulin and they soon become insulin resistant. For those who are parents, it's like a child constantly shouting loudly into your ear, eventually you just stop listening, even if the house is on fire.

That's exactly what happens to your cells. They stop listening to the message of insulin to take your excess sugar and store it as glycogen and as a result your sugar gets stored as fat.

How To Create A High Metabolism That Burns Fat Not Sugar

When most experts talk about increasing your metabolism, the question is whether you are increasing your metabolism to burn sugar or to burn fat. For that reason there is an important distinction to be made because you want to be concerned with the quality of your metabolism and not just the quantity.

The goal is to create a high metabolism that burns fat because a sugar-burning metabolism is just way too much work and leads to very little results. This is the reason why many people keep working out day after day for weeks on end without any results.

The goal is not just to increase your metabolism, but to turn your body into a fat burner. You want your body to turn to your fat stores and not to sugar for a majority of your activities. As a result, you will lose weight and feel good without the fatigue of dragging yourself to the gym for hours on end.

Sugar slams the emergency brakes on the amount of fat your body will burn. It's not just a matter of calories in vs. calories out - it's a double whammy. You stop burning fat and start storing what you have eaten as fat.

Tip #1: Know How Much

Know how much sugar you should consume, as this number is different for everyone. Take your goal weight, divide by 10, and then add 10 and that is the maximum amount of sugar you want to consume daily. So for example if your goal weight is 150 pounds, take 150 and divide that by 10 which is 15 then add 10 which is a total of 25 and 25 grams is your maximum amount of sugar you want to consume daily.

Get out a calculator now and find your ideal sugar intake.

Tip #2: Be A Food Detective

Start reading your labels and see how much sugar you're consuming. Sugar is listed in grams. The accompanying picture shows a nutrition label from a bottle of Gatorade. Note the serving size and servings per container. Most folks think that Gatorade and other sugar loaded energy drinks are good for you. I have news for you, they are not, unless you are a highly tuned athlete who competes at the national level and are in dire need of sugar as a quick fix to increase athletic performance.

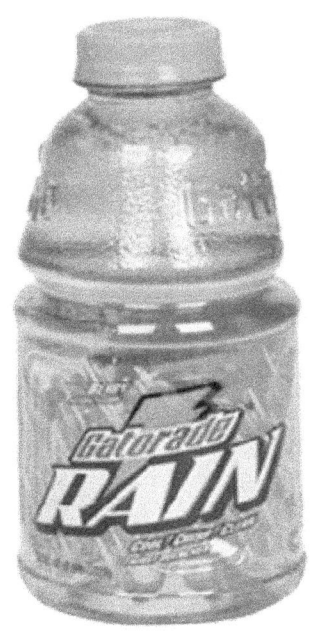

Nutrition Facts

Serving Size 8 fl oz (240ml)
Servings Per Container 4

Amount Per Serving

Calories 50

	% Daily Value*
Total Fat 0g	0%
Sodium 110mg	5%
Potassium 30mg	1%
Total Carbohydrate 14g	5%
Sugars 14g	
Protein 0g	

Not a significant source of Calories From Fat, Saturated Fat, Cholesterol, Dietary Fiber, Vitamin A, Vitamin C, Calcium, Iron.

* Percent Daily Values are based on a 2,000 calorie diet.

Let's examine the label. It says it's only 50 calories, but if we take a deeper look, it has 14 grams of sugar per serving size. This bottle has 4 servings which means if you drink the entire bottle, you will be consuming a total of 56 grams of sugar.

Remember our 150 pound person example? Their daily sugar intake should be no more than 25 grams. If this person had this bottle of Gatorade, they would already have doubled their sugar requirement.

Tip #3: There Is No Value In Super Sizing.

We've all been tricked, even when we thought we were being smart. You are told a slice of cake costs $3, but the entire cake consisting of 100 slices costs $6. *As a result, you start thinking with your wallet instead of your waist!* Buying the entire cake is not a good deal, just as buying half a trunk full of soda and juice is not a good deal. It's just a cheaper way to add more sugar and therefore more fat to your body.

When you hear about super sizing, remember they are referring to your waist size and not to food value.

Tip #4: Being Aware

You need to be aware and on guard at those times when your sugar cravings will hit you, and they will. Remember cravings are momentary and you want to choose healthier alternatives. However just by following some of the strategies in this program, you will encounter much fewer sugar cravings. Nevertheless, you still need to be totally aware of those times when you experience them.

Be Aware of Exhaustion

Be aware that if you are sleep deprived or exhausted, your body often thinks its tiredness is a result of low blood sugar. Your brain signals your body to start craving sugar or carbohydrates.

Be Aware of Stress

When you are constantly under stress, your adrenal glands secrete adrenaline, which makes your body very responsive to a stressful environment. But once adrenaline starts dwindling down, your energy level will automatically drop significantly, causing you to crave a quick source of energy.

Be Aware of Hormonal Changes

For women, just before menstruation, when estrogen is low and beta-endorphin levels are at their lowest, craving for sugar can seem unmanageable.

Men are not exempt from hormonal changes as there is a syndrome known as Irritable male syndrome (IMS), described as a state of hypersensitivity, being easily frustrated, anxious and unrelenting anger. All these symptoms are associated with biochemical changes, male hormonal fluctuations and yes, food cravings.

Tip #5: Make Better Decisions While Shopping

Make the right choices while shopping. Not all carbs are created equal. You want more whole grain, unrefined products. Moderate your use of highly processed and refined carbs found in most white breads, flours, white rice, pastas and breakfast cereals.

Tip #6: Eat Good Fat

We will talk more about this in the alkalinity and acidic module, but eat good fat. It's impossible to lose weight without eating good fats. Eating fat does not make you fat and when you eat the right kind of fat your body begins to burn even the unwanted fat.

Nature's Cure vs. Manufacturers' Deception

It's perfectly normal to have a sweet tooth and the reason nature designed it this way is to make us love eating veggies and fruits. Why? Because they are such a goldmine of vitamins, minerals and fiber. However since food manufacturers know of this weakness, they have exploited our desire for sweets by making everything sweet.

The sweetness in fruits is a type of sugar called fructose. In nature when you find fructose you will find fiber in mass because *when nature creates a poison it also creates an antidote.* This means that the natural fiber found in fruits will help reduce the rate of the sugar absorption and also increase the rate of satiety so you feel full faster.

That's why it's easy to drink a glass of orange juice (which has up to five oranges in one glass) in just a few minutes than it is to actually eat those five oranges. Seriously, when was that last time you ate five oranges in one sitting?

Some people think that smoothies or fruit juices are better, but some of them have 99 grams worth of sugar. Remember, your body was not meant to eat that much sugar in one sitting.

12 ounces of >>>>>>>	Coca-Cola	Orange Juice	Apple Juice	Cherry Juice	Grape Juice
Total carbohydrates	40 g	39 g	42 g	49.5 g	60 g
Carbs from sugar	40 g	33 g	39 g	37.5 g	58.5 g
Sugar (teaspoons)	10 tsp	8 tsp	10 tsp	9 tsp	15 tsp
Calories	145	165	165	210	240

There is absolutely no reason you should regularly drink fruit juices regardless of how organic or natural they are. All the vitamins and minerals you need are in the actual fruit. If nature wanted you to drink the orange juice, it would have made it hollow so all you did was pop in a straw and drink up.

My simple advice: if you want to lose weight and burn fat, you want to wean yourself off drinking fruit juices, or just dilute them if you can't completely stop. For many just this simple tip will result in 10 pounds or more of weight loss in just a few weeks.

Alternative Sweeteners

You might be thinking that alternative sweeteners are a solution to your sugar problem, but not the ones that most are familiar with. Examples of common alternative sweeteners are

Saccharin – Usually packaged as Sweet N Low
Aspartame – Packaged as Equal and NutraSweet
Sucralose – Packaged as Splenda
HFC – High fructose corn syrup.

You can get away with them if you have them in small amounts like in chewing gum but please limit your intake if you consume them in large quantities like in diet sodas. For some having large amounts of these alternative sweeteners can be worse than the effects of sugar.

Also other natural sweeteners such as honey, sugar beets, or agave nectar have the same effect as sugar in the blood and are therefore not helpful.

Using Smart and Safe Sugars

Use instead what I call smart and safe sugars. If you want something healthy that can give you a real sweet taste, use my list of recommended sugar alcohols or another natural sweetener called stevia.

Sugar Alcohols

There are several kinds of sugar alcohols but the most common are xylitol, maltitol and erythritol, which can all be found online or at most health food stores and some grocery stores.

Please don't be deceived by the classification 'sugar alcohols' because these are neither sugar nor alcoholic, but rather are a type of carbohydrate that is not fully absorbed by the body. As a result, these do not cause blood sugar spikes and are eliminated from the body through urine.

Xylitol - The first and probably most popular sugar alcohol. It's found in the fibers of many fruits and vegetables.

Maltitol - Another popular sugar alcohol that has close to 90% the identical properties of table sugar, but has fewer calories. Commercially you will find it under names such as **Maltisorb** and **Maltisweet.**

Erythritol - One of the better sugar alcohols to use. It occurs naturally in fruits and fermented foods. It's almost non-caloric and is 60–70% as sweet as table sugar with almost no effect on blood sugar. It is absorbed by the body and less likely to cause gastric side effects like other sugar alcohols can.

Stevia

The other sweetener is not a sugar alcohol but a leaf extract called Stevia. On food labels you will find it identified scientifically as Stevia rebaudiana. Stevia is a natural herb and its extracts are 300 times the sweetness of sugar, with a negligible effect on blood sugar.

Usually in drop form, a little stevia goes a long way. If you put too much in your coffee, it's overwhelming. I personally use it and like it, but some think it has a slight aftertaste. Studies have shown that stevia may be effective in reducing hypertension, aka. high blood pressure.

Stevia has also been shown to improve insulin sensitivity and possibly even to promote additional insulin production to help reverse diabetes and metabolic syndrome.

Pruvia and Truvia

The beverage industry has joined the bandwagon too. Sometime in early 2009, Coca-Cola and Cargill released Truvia and Pruvia.

These sweeteners have three ingredients: stevia, erythritol, and natural flavors – whatever that means. Despite my written requests and phone calls, the companies have refused to say exactly what the third ingredient is. All they say is that it's proprietary (top secret). It's used to improve the taste and bulk it up.

I'm always wary of proprietary or secret blends by food manufacturers, so I don't give them my 100% endorsement. However, they appear safe for use.

Fiber – Natures Sugar Cure
Eat More Fiber

The quickest and best way to improve your diet without making a lot of changes is to add more fiber. Eating more fiber with your meals is your winning lottery ticket to a slimmer and healthier you.

Fiber comes from fruits, vegetables, grains, nuts and legumes. It's a type of carbohydrate that your body cannot digest. Fiber can't be broken down or absorbed into the bloodstream and contains no calories. Fiber simply passes through the entire digestive tract, but this does not mean it has no value for you.

Dietary fiber will give you that feeling of early satisfaction in a meal so it makes you feel full faster and for much longer. This means you are less likely to be hungry a couple of hours after eating. Fiber will help you eat less food, less often and the reduction in calories will help you lose weight.

Fiber is important because it slows down digestion in the stomach and small intestine, thereby helping to stabilize blood sugar levels. This means that eating fiber reduces sugar spikes in your body. The sugar is absorbed much more slowly and over a period of time. Nature is pretty smart too because wherever you find natural sweetness, you find fiber.

Most folks eat about 10 grams of fiber or less a day and in reality we need 40 grams or more. Your goal is to add more fiber to your meals which is easier than you think.

I enjoy eating blackberries and raspberries as a way to get my fiber. Did you know that a single cup of these berries has about 8 grams of fiber? All I do is add them to my breakfast.

I really like avocados. They are very nutritious with so much goodness in them: For example a medium avocado has 14 grams of fiber.

Pinto beans include 8 grams of fiber in ½ a cup and they're easy to add to many recipes.

When I cook my rice, I will add sliced raw almonds which include 4 grams of fiber per ounce.

Here are some additional ways you can eat more fiber:
1. Eat more of the whole fruits than drinking just fruit juice. Eat the orange rather than drinking orange juice.
2. Eat the skins of apples and pears and don't peel your potatoes. The skin can add 10 grams of fiber to your diet every day.
3. Eat whole-grain versions of your foods, rather than refined grains. Choose 100% whole grain breads instead of refined breads.
4. Add more veggies to your stews or soup.
5. Eat beans and other legumes such as peas and lentils a few times a week.
6. Eat more raw nuts, such as almonds, cashews, macadamia and Brazil nuts which are rich in fiber and healthy fats.

Module 2: Summary

Eat more fiber and consume less sugar. Be mindful of the sugar you consume.

For extra credit, use the formula of dividing your goal weight by 10 then adding 10 and use that for the maximum amount of sugar you consume per day.

At a bare minimum, try cutting back on drinking fruit juices regardless of whether they are 100% juice. It's not a good idea to drink your calories regardless of what promises they make. They still have a ton of sugar. Yes the vitamins and minerals are in there too, but the sugar without the natural fiber completely halts your chances of burning fat.

Eat the whole fruit instead. If you have to drink juices, reduce the amount or dilute with water. Also be careful with your deserts, cakes, chocolate and all the usual sugary suspects.

MODULE 3

Alkalinity and Water

Your Body's Acid and Alkaline Balance

How acidic you are determines so much about your health, including how much fat your body stores and how much it will want to let go.

Environment Is Everything

In life, we have to create the right environment for anything good to happen. Imagine you have a very important paper to write. Can you envision doing this at a rock concert? Regardless of how hard you concentrate, you will not be able to focus on what you are doing.

In the same way, we have to create an environment to burn fat. Regardless of how much you exercise or what supplements you take, if the environment is not conducive to health and fat burning, you are basically driving while stepping on both the brake and the gas pedals.

Just as if you throw seeds on a concrete floor, no matter how good the seeds are and how often you water them, they will not flourish. The environment is everything and the right environment for your body begins with the right pH balance. It's one of the most important measurements of health and important for those who want to burn fat.

Over Acid = Over Fat

Most people are surprised to find it's not they are over-fat, but they are over-acid because if your blood is overly acidic, you will tend to store fat regardless of how much you exercise for two reasons. First, your body holds on to the fat because fat helps protect your organs and tissues from the deadly effects of too much acid in the body. Secondly, if you are too acidic, the overall effectiveness of hormones such as insulin, glucagon and growth hormone which control the amount of fat you burn is greatly reduced.

The Basics Of pH

So what is pH? For those who are able to recall a little 5th grade science the abbreviation stands for "potential for hydrogen" and is a measurement of the concentration of hydrogen ions in solutions. It's what is used to measure the acidity or alkalinity of a substance. In case you're wondering, sometimes instead of alkaline some will say 'base' or 'basic,' but it all means the same thing.

pH is a scale ranging from values of 0 to 14. If a substance is a 7, it means it's perfectly neutral. Numbers below 7 are acidic and the numbers above 7 are alkaline or bases.

The perfect pH for the human blood is a pH of 7.365. You will notice that it's slightly alkaline. If the pH goes to 7.2, you will die that's how delicate the balance is. Remember your body's primary role is survival so it tries its best to keep you in that perfect pH balance by making adjustments. Often these adjustments by your body result in numerous health problems including storing fat.

There are many ways to measure your pH. Of course, measurement of your blood pH is the most accurate and your doctor can send your blood to the lab for those who need concrete evidence. You can also test your urine and saliva in the morning with special pH test strips available at your local pharmacy. This will not be entirely accurate, but it will give you a good idea of where you are.

Food pH

There is a difference between the pH of a specific food you consume and its effect on your body. Some foods are very acidic like lemons and limes, but they have an alkaline effect on your body. So adding fresh lemon or lime juice to your water will help alkalize your body.

Remember, anything you consume has to be assimilated then or eliminated. When you eat food, it's metabolized in the body but it will always leave behind a residue or ash. The pH of the food is shown by its ash or its residue after it has gone through the digestive process. If the residue is more acidic, then it will lessen the alkalinity of the blood. If the residue is more alkaline, then your blood becomes more alkaline and it will increase your resistance to diseases, help you burn fat and lose weight.

Remember, environment is critical for anything to happen.

To understand this, one must come to the realization that neutralizing acid is not a 1 to 1 ratio. It takes 20 parts of alkalinity to neutralize 1 part of acid. So when your body gets acidic, it will sacrifice parts of itself to get back to an alkaline state.

Your body will "borrow" minerals and nutrients such as calcium and magnesium from bones and even other minerals such as potassium and sodium from your organs.

The #1 thing that is responsible for the biggest breakdown in the body is acidity. You become really prone to fatigue and illnesses and have low bone density. More cholesterol is released in the system to protect the body and the organs from the acid, and the body creates more body fat to protect itself.

In an acidic environment, you will be prone to inflammation, joint pain, fungus overgrowth, immune dysfunction, and - this might come as a shock to many – cancer, which will only thrive in an acidic environment.

There are many alkaline courses that give you so many restrictions but my goal is to make it easy and practical for you. So the most important thing for us is to moderate acidic foods.

Now you cannot entirely avoid all of the acidic foods I will list, but if you are going to consume them, do it in moderation. Going from one extreme to another is a big contributor to yo-yo dieting. Rather than eliminate, moderate. A little bit of your favorite foods no matter how unhealthy you think they are, will take you a long way. It will help your psyche so you don't feel deprived and prevent you from going on a binge.

Alkalizing Your Body - Foods To Moderate
Milk in Moderation

Here is a big problem: milk. One of the biggest myths is that milk is good for strong bones. This is the furthest thing away from the truth. In fact, the excessive consumption of dairy products creates bone loss.

Yes, milk does contain calcium but consuming too much of it actually creates an environment in the body that leaches calcium from your bones. So it's not more calcium we need but we need to stop the body from losing it. Think about it, when the Titanic hit the iceberg, what was more important, pumping the water out or stopping the damage by plugging the hole?

Got Milk?

The dairy industry tries to get you to drink more milk through lobbying and advertising. Who do you think makes those milk commercials? Follow the money, they can say whatever they want to say in advertising. Look this up: the countries with the highest rates of osteoporosis are the ones where people drink the most milk such as the U.S., England, and Sweden. Coincidence? Absolutely not.

The Heist

A bank manager should not celebrate when he sees five guys with ski masks and huge duffel bags walk into a bank pretending to be customers. They are faking being customers because they are there to rob the bank. Yes, milk has a lot of calcium but it's not what you are drinking but what happens at the end of your drinking milk. If you drink too much milk, your body will lose calcium in the process.

Cow's milk will turn a 70 pound calf at birth into a 1200 pound cow in just a year. Does that seem like something you want to do with your body? I don't think so.

Instead of drinking a lot of cow's milk, opt for almond milk. My favorite brand is Almond Breeze and it's available at most grocery stores. I will take it when I drink my morning tea and also with my oatmeal.

Should you completely avoid milk and its products? Well your body can handle it in moderation. Just don't drink it like its water, thinking you are doing your body a favor.

Sugar In Moderation

Just like in the Sugar and Fiber modules, the amount of sugar you consume is a major contributor to increased acidity in your body. The extra sugar that cannot be burned or stored is fermented into acids. Everything in the insulin and sugar module applies here, especially avoiding fruit juices and soft drinks like the plague (because they are a plague). You might not realize this but one of the key ingredients in colas is phosphoric acid that has a pH level of 2.5.

Animal Protein in Moderation

Digestion is the most underestimated human function. The pharmaceutical companies know most people think of it as a bother and sales of gastroin-testinal remedies are one of the largest profit margins in the pharmaceuti-cal business.

The body does not mess around with digestion because all our major organs play a role in digestion. A healthy digestive system almost always means you are in good health. If you lack energy, you can often trace it back to what's happening in your digestive process, or what's NOT happening.

We were designed to eat meat in moderation and not with every single meal. Of course, the beef industry says otherwise. Beef is what's for dinner, right? The truth is that we are not carnivores. Real carnivores have jaws that can easily slide for a good grip when they bite and big sharp canine teeth for removing meat from the body. For humans, all of our teeth are about the same height and our canines are projected only a little bit and our jaws basically just go up and down.

A real carnivore's intestinal tract is short relative to the length of their body so when they eat meat, it travels quickly in and out of the body. When we eat a lot of meat, our digestive system is not as quick and the meat will putrefy inside of us. This is similar to what happens when you leave meat outside. It begins to turn purple and blue.

High consumption of meat will make the body acidic and consumption of red meat has been associated with increased osteoporosis, colon cancer, prostate cancer, and breast cancer cases. Is that what you want to have for dinner?

Instead, you want to moderate eating the meats of all the four-legged ani-mals or consume them sparingly. I enjoy a good steak like anyone, but it's not every day. Some weeks I go without eating meat, and most of the time it's 2 – 3 times per week that I indulge in some sort of animal product.

If you are going to eat meat, make some good choices. Animals were designed to eat grass but unfortunately most industrialized nations food systems are based on grains and as a result most of our grain fed cattle are obese. In addition hormones and antibiotics are added to help them handle the consumption of grains. And where do those chemicals go? Onto your dinner plate.

If you are going to eat meat, be smart. Make sure it's hormone free and has no antibiotics. For beef, try to make sure the cows were grass fed and raised ethically.

How About Chicken?

Chicken is a slightly better option. Slightly.

If you are going to eat chicken, just like beef, make sure it is hormone and antibiotic free, raised in a cage free environment and on a vegetarian organic diet, like flax seed.

The general idea, is that the less legs in the animal the better. Fish (which we will cover later) is better than chicken and chicken is better than beef.

All in all, for good health, I recommend a couple of days in a week where you don't eat beef or chicken and focus on getting more fruits, vegetables, beans and nuts in your meals instead of meat.

Don't I Need A Lot of Protein?

But what happens if you moderate the amount of meat you eat? Will you get enough protein? It's an argument you hear over and over. Most people eat way too much meat and the beef industry has all the money in the world to protect its interests. Just ask Oprah who was sued for talking negatively about meat.

What most people don't know is that all the amino acids that you need for your body to make high quality protein are from plant sources – all of them.

The healthiest and strongest animals in the world such as horses, gorillas, and elephants all eat plants. You don't see them go for protein shakes or meat.

Dave Scott is not only a six-time Ironman Champion but also a vegetarian! Ironman is the ultimate endurance test: A 2.4 mile swim, 112 mile bike ride, and a 26.2 mile marathon which all have to be done in less than 17 hours. Yes, vegetarians still get the protein they need.

Alcohol In Moderation

Alcohol in few words is toxic. When you consume alcohol, fat burning and other vital body functions are put on hold. Your body, in order to survive has to get rid of the alcohol through all channels. Your breath, sweat, bowels are all employed to detoxify your body. Drinking alcohol moderately has a place in society, but frequently drinking alcohol, whether its beer or wine, will make you fat.

Alcohol is basically fermented sugar. Not only do you get the damaging effects of alcohol on the body, but your body will metabolize the alcohol into fat, plus all the byproducts of alcohol metabolism are very acidic to the body. I would encourage you to avoid daily drinking and weekend binge drinking. Choose instead, to have a drink or two every now and then. And for every drink, have a glass of water to help with the detoxification.

Guidelines For Alkaline Foods

So what are alkaline forming foods? You ask. The goal of this course was not to give you recipes or a specific list of foods, but to give you general guidelines for making your own decisions.

Don't get hang up in wanting a specific list of foods to eat, if you adhere to the guidelines below, a whole world of options will open up to you and getting alkaline will not feel restrictive. Generally speaking, alkaline forming foods are foods in their raw and natural state like fruits and veggies. Below you will find my recommendations of foods and supplements that will increase your alkalinity.

What To Eat In Abundance
Eat more Vegetables

Nothing really new here but what you need to know is that veggies can provide most of the body's vitamins, minerals, and fiber. Additionally, green vegetables contain chlorophyll. Chlorophyll is what gives plants their green color and is particularly important to you because it is very similar to human blood in both chemical and molecular structure. The phytonutrients in plants, which also give them the yellow, red, and orange colors, will help neutralize acid in your body and act as antioxidants. Some of my favorite, very alkalizing foods are tomatoes (uncooked), avocado, spinach, and broccoli.

Eat More FAT

Please don't be fooled about the low fat craze right now - it's misleading. The diet industry truly began in 1982 when the American Heart Association (AHA), American Medical Association (AMA), and USDA cautioned us to reduce total fat consumption from 40% to 30%.

Surprisingly, we have done just that. Fat consumption is down, but we have more obese people, more diabetes and more heart problems than ever. **It's not the fat.** This recommendation is the main reason we are all fatter than we ever have been.

Accumulating fat is not about eating fat, but about sugar. Fat is not the enemy you should be afraid of. In fact, a recent Mayo Clinic study followed women on a high fat diet who then switched to a low fat diet. Researchers found there was no change in their weight loss.

This low fat craze has caused a chain reaction that is at the heart of the current problem with the diet industry. Fat makes everything taste better. So when the food manufacturers remove fat from their foods, the taste and flavor disappear. As a result, the companies add sugar.

We need to eat fat, especially good fat because the more good fat we eat, the more we increase our ability to burn body fat.

Eat good fats – Fats are your friend

To lose weight, you must consume and increase the amount of quality fat in your diet. You heard it right: eat more fat. This is counterintuitive for most of us, because of all the low fat nonsense that gets preached to us.

Good fats are one of the most important foods you will eat that can regulate your weight. Here's why you need to be eating more good fat.

Reason 1: Eating Good Fat Will Buffer or Neutralize Acid

Your body uses fat to buffer or neutralize acids. Eating the right amounts of fat will allow the fat to bind with excess acids and eliminate them from the body, helping you lose weight more easily.

Reason 2: Eating Good Fat Helps You Burn Body Fat

Most people burn sugar for fuel, but, given a chance, the body will burn fat. Fat is a slower, but much cleaner fuel that uses less energy and produces way less acid in the process. It's the body's greenest fuel because it creates 5 times more energy than burning sugar. Think about that: it's like your car going from 20 mpg to 100 mpg, minus all the harmful emissions. Eating fat helps you burn off the excess body fat you have accumulated.

Reason 3: Eating Good Fat Controls Your Appetite

Eating good fat will help you lose weight because good fats will regulate your appetite. Fat slows down the rate at which food gets emptied out of the stomach; this means you will feel more full after a meal, feel less hungry between meals and have fewer cravings.

Reason 4: Few Insulin Spikes – More Fat Burning

Fat will slow down the rate of sugar absorbed in the small intestines; this will keep insulin secretions low and help you burn more fat.

What Types of Fat To Avoid

My goal is to make it simple, rather than give you a doctoral dissertation on the different types of fats.

Avoid Trans Fat

The trans fats we are talking about are artificially made trans fats. Although small amounts of trans fat occur naturally in some meat and dairy products, it's the trans fats in processed foods that seem to be more harmful.

Trans fats are made by adding hydrogen to vegetable oil through a process called hydrogenation. Trans fats are more solid than oil is, making them less likely to spoil. Using trans fats in the manufacturing of foods helps foods stay fresh longer and have a longer shelf life with a less greasy feel.

Trans fats really give fat a bad name and are the worst because of their impact on your cholesterol levels. Unlike other fats, trans fats — also called trans-fatty acids — both raise your "bad" (LDL) cholesterol and lower your "good" (HDL) cholesterol. These fats will impair your blood circulation and increase the risk of many degenerative diseases.

Trans fats used to be more common, but in recent years, food manufacturers have used them less because of concerns over the health effects. In fact, their use is banned in a few states.

While it's good that trans fats are being listed on labels, you should be aware of what nutritional labels really mean when it comes to trans fat. For example, if a food has less than 0.5 grams of trans fat per serving, the food label can read 0 grams trans fat. Though that's a small amount of trans fat, if you eat multiple servings of foods with less than 0.5 grams of trans fat, you could exceed recommended limits.

So become a food detective and read your food labels. How do you know whether food contains trans fat? Look for the words "partially hydrogenated" or hydrogenated oil. Also look out for the word "shortening" as shortening includes some trans fats.

Good Fats to consume

Flaxseed Oil
Extra Virgin Olive Oil
Almond Oil
Avocado Oil
Refined Walnut Oil
Sesame seeds and Sesame Oils
Safflower Oil
Coconut Oil

Best Way To Consume Your Fat

The best way to consume your fat is to take your food fats in oil form. Take about 2 to 4 tablespoons of oil every day on an empty stomach at least

3 hours after your last meal and then wait about 30 minutes to an hour before eating. This way, your body can use it immediately and process it without trying to break down other foods.

I find taking my tablespoons of oil in the morning very convenient. Everyone's stomach reacts differently to oil so find out which one works best for you.

The best oils to drink are

1. Refined Walnut Oil
2. Extra Virgin Olive Oil
3. Flaxseed Oil

So start with 1 tablespoon for a couple of days and then upgrade to 2 tablespoons. Then after about a month or so you can add a 3rd tablespoon.

Water – Essence of Life

If you don't drink water, you will get fat. Many folks mistake thirst for hunger and if you are hungry and tired, 9 out of 10 times it's because you are dehydrated.

Water is essential for everything in the body. When I say everything, I mean everything. There is nothing in the body that does not require the involvement of water.

Your body is 75% water. Over 75% of your muscle is water, 80% of your brain is water, 95% of your eyes, 85% of your kidneys, and even 25% of your bones contain water. It's the reason when a body is cremated it can fit into a little urn.

The problem most nutritionists make is to focus on food, but if the body is 75% water and 25% solid isn't it more important to focus on what we drink rather than what we eat? Think about that.

In order for the body to survive, you have to have oxygen. Without it, you will be dead in a few minutes. The next important thing is not food because we can survive without food for weeks, but the most important nutrient after oxygen is water, because without it we would be dead in a matter of days.

So how much water should you consume? Drink half your weight or target weight in ounces as a minimum. So, if you weigh 150 pounds, half of that in ounces would be 75 ounces of water. And don't just gulp all if it down at once. Yes, you can down a glass here and there, but sip the rest slowly throughout the day.

As we get older, our thirst seems to fade away. For those who are over 50 or approaching it, you might be nodding your head right now. The reason you are not as thirsty as you used to be is that your body's thirst sensation has diminished and will continue diminishing with age. You might suffer symptoms of dehydration such as muscle cramps (especially leg cramps), dizziness, decreased vision, mental confusion or lack of mental clarity, heart palpitations, and more.

If you drink more water, yes just water, you will dramatically slow down your aging. Here are my recommendations on the kinds of water to drink.

Eat Your Water

Packaged by mother nature, life's perfect water is alive and is contained in high water content foods. These are your fruits and veggies and most of them are 90% water content and above. The water in these foods is fresh and easier for the body to absorb and you even don't have to think about it. You get to hydrate yourself while eating at the same time.

Drink Filtered Water

Drink filtered water because if you don't filter your water, your body will need to act as the filter. I use the Zero water filter which is one of the very few filters available in the market that removes 100% of detectable dissolved solids in water and meets the FDA's definition for purified bottled water. However, if this is not available where you are, get any other water filter because something is better than nothing.

Please try to avoid drinking bottled water as much as possible unless you don't have another option. First, the impact to the environment is staggering, and second almost half of the water that is currently bottled is actually tap water. Also most of the plastic bottles contain a chemical called bisphenol A or BPA that is been linked to many serious health problems.

Alkalize Your Water

Increasing the alkalinity of your water is highly recommended. After you filter water, try to increase the pH of your water. There are three ways to do this.

1. Use pH Drops. I get mine from Amazon.com. Just search for 'alkazone ph drops." I've included a picture. There are several brands coming out, each with lots of benefits. It's best to research what works best for you.

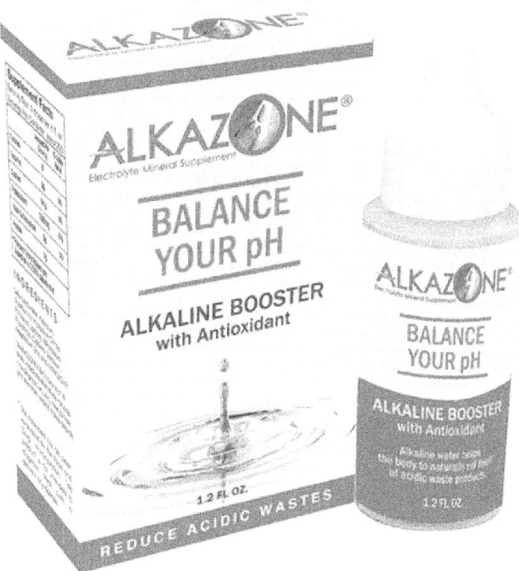

2. Squeeze lemon or lime juice into your water. How easy can it get?
3. You can also add alkaline salts that you can buy from most health food stores and add them to your water: sodium bicarbonate, magnesium bicarbonate, or calcium bicarbonate.

I prefer to get the drops, add them to my filtered water, and I'm good to go.

Drink More Green Drinks

This is the easiest and best way to alkalize your body. Normally, I will drink 2-3 glasses of a green drink every day. Every 4 to 6 months when I want to detoxify my body, I will drink at least half my body weight in ounces of green drink.

The easiest way is to buy concentrated and powdered greens and all you have to do is mix them with water. Green drinks are not smoothies, but a blend of highly alkaline grasses and mostly green vegetables that are full of chlorophyll in powdered form. Examples of these powdered greens are wheat grass, barley grass, and other powdered vegetables. A teaspoon of your green powdered drinks is the equivalent to a pound of fresh veggies. Can you imagine getting all your vegetables in one drink?

Green drinks are very alkalizing, super nutritious, and they have chlorophyll, which deserves a special mention because it's nature's most powerful blood detoxifier and builder.

If you consume chlorophyll, not only will you be building and cleansing your blood, but you will be strengthening your immune system and helping to get rid of unhealthy bacteria.

Chlorophyll Is Similar To Blood

The reason chlorophyll is such an effective blood builder and cleanser is that chemically speaking, chlorophyll is very similar to the hemoglobin found in the red blood cells.

The only difference is that the red blood cells have iron as the center atom whereas chlorophyll has magnesium. This similarity makes it very easy for the body to create new red blood cells from chlorophyll.

My favorite brand of wheat grass is called Amazing Grass Organic Wheat Grass Powder by Amazing Grass. I buy the bigger 17-ounce container. You can buy it at your favorite health food store or buy it from Amazon as I do. Below is a picture.

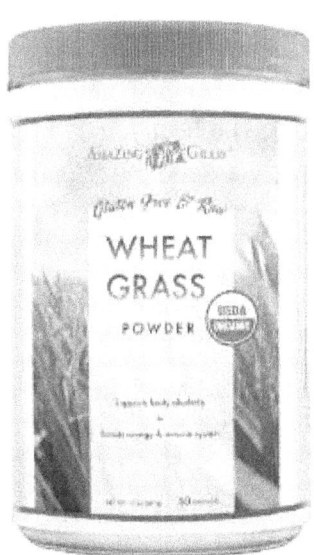

Module 3: Summary

If you want to lose fat and still be healthy, you must consume good fat. So embrace good fat as part of your lifestyle. Start with 1 tablespoon for a couple of days and then upgrade to 2 tablespoons. Then after about a month or so, you can add a 3rd tablespoon. Remember, it's best to take your oil on an empty stomach at least 3 hours after your last meal and 30 minutes to an hour or so before eating. I find mornings work best, but it's your personal preference.

The three best fats you can drink include:
1. Refined Walnut Oil
2. Extra Virgin Olive Oil
3. Flaxseed Oil.

For extra credit and even better results, buy yourself some wheat grass from your health food store or from online shops. I personally like to buy from Amazon.com

Make sure to drink filtered water, at least half your body weight in ounces, all throughout during the day. The best you can really do is to buy a water bottle that you can easily carry around the house, in the office or wherever life takes you.

MODULE 4

Short and Intermittent Fasting

Main Reason For Weight Loss

When you take in less than you burn off through your metabolism or activity, you lose weight. That's it. We can debate all the other stuff, but think about how many times you've heard conflicting and confusing new studies about different diet recommendations.

The truth is that most of the current research on diet and nutrition is not to improve our health and wellness, but is a cleverly disguised marketing gimmick dressed up as science.

Even though some people are able to lose weight on many different diet programs, the problem is that these diets can be very restrictive and cannot be sustained. As you have discovered, they are very few hardcore restrictions with my program. My goal is to provide you with a blueprint for long term health and weight loss without suffocating you with a lot of do's and don'ts.

The techniques I will describe in this module are probably the easiest and most effective things you can do for your long term health and well-being. Listen up now because a few recommendations from this chapter will allow you to continue eating most of the foods you enjoy but still lose weight and to keep it off.

Misinformation About Frequency of Food

The problem we face is that much of the misinformation has been propagated by the food industry. Their goal is to always keep us eating to improve their sales and profits.

Let's look at the myth that for you to boost your metabolism, you have to eat six times a day. Now for a moment step into my common sense corner and ask the obvious question, do you think that's how our bodies were designed to eat?

Think about our primitive ancestors. Once the animal they had caught or the fruits and berries they had gathered were eaten, they had to go searching for more food. Do you think they ate six times a day? Of course not. They did not even eat three meals a day. Do you think they skipped meals? All the time.

Our Bodies Need A Break

Our bodies were designed to eat and then take a break. That is the beauty of the design. Everything in your body is designed to take a break, even if your boss doesn't think so.

Most people think that your heart is working all the time – not so. What you don't realize is that the heart is actually resting for 70-80% of the time. It beats, takes a much longer rest then beats again. This is how it keeps us alive and pumps blood to all parts of the body.

You breathe in and out. Your muscles contract and relax. There is rest designed everywhere in your body and once a while, you should give your digestive system a rest.

What is the digestive system?

The digestive system is all the way from your mouth to your behind and everything in between. It's very energy intensive and a major player in the human body.

Here is a funny story. It's said when God made the body, different parts of the body were arguing who was going to be the boss. The brain explained that since it controlled everything, it should be boss. The legs said, "I take the body everywhere it wants to go. I should be boss." The eyes said, "I see everything, I should be the boss." Then the anus applied for the job but the other parts of the body found this suggestion ridiculous and laughed so hard. So much so that the butt hole become mad and closed up!

After a few days, the brain went foggy, the legs got wobbly, the eyes got crossed, and they all agreed that they should make the anus the boss.

Make sense?

Well, there is a punch line about the kind of person it takes to be a boss but that's not my point. My goal is to highlight how important your entire digestive tract is.

Take A Digestive Vacation!

The digestive system works very hard for you behind the scenes. In the lifetime of the average person, this series of organs will process about 30 tons of food. Don't you think it needs a break?

The body was designed to eat then fast, but you will not hear this being promoted anywhere. The food and beverage industry knows that people eating less is bad for business. So they spend millions of dollars in lobbying the government, millions of dollars in funding research groups, and they spend close to 40 billion of dollars (that's with a B) in advertising.

All you will hear are different ways to eat more: six meals per day, high protein, lots of high calcium foods, etc. But what you will not hear from the food industry is "learn how to take a break from eating, because it does your body a lot of good"

The government does not really want to tell you to take a break from eating because it's bad for the economy. If they ever had the guts to do it, you would see unprecedented lobbying, advertising, and even lawsuits from the food and beverage industry.

Fasting Is In Most Cultures and Religions

You were not designed to eat all the time. Our bodies were designed to fast and this is an idea embraced by many different cultures and religions. Most religions have some sort of fasting built into their rites and rituals. Why? Because there is a lot of magic that happens when your body is in a state of fasting.

When you get sick, the first thing your body does is kill your appetite. You can drink, but you definitely don't want to anything eat. Why do you think this is the case?

Because the process of absorbing, using, and then eliminating food is very energy intensive. All the body's major organs are called upon – it's all hands on deck. Your brain, kidney, liver, pancreas, etc. have to get involved at one time or another.

When you are not feeling well, the body needs to get rid of toxins created by your illness. It then has to heal and repair itself and it cannot do that when you are stuffed. Since digestion takes a lot of vital energy and too many resources, the decision gets made for you. If you fall sick – you have no appetite. This gives the body the vital chance to clean house. The body can only heal and repair itself in the 'fasted state'.

You already fast every day

Think about sleep which is basically your daily fast. The word we use for the first meal of the day is made up of two words that mean to break your fast. Sleep is your body's highest anabolic state, where it repairs, grows, and rejuvenates the immune, nervous, skeletal, and muscular systems.

Unfortunately, what you will come across is a lot of misinformation on fasting, all of it ridiculous and highly exaggerated. Some say fasting damages your metabolism or eats up your muscles – such nonsense! None of this will happen with short and flexible fasting.

Short and Flexible Fasting Defined

Short and flexible fasting is willingly planning to go without some food for a pre-determined period of time.

It's important to note the words **willingly** and **pre-determined** because it indicates that you are planning for it, which is critical.

My formula for flexible and short term fasting is twofold.
1. Have the time between your first meal and last meal be about 11-12 hours. Allow about 12 hours between dinner and breakfast.
2. Fast once or twice a week for 20 – 24 hours.

The beauty about short and flexible fasting is that you still get to eat every single day.

Short and flexible fasting is about giving your body a much needed vacation from the rigors of digestion.

Avoid Snacking – Instead Eat Real Meals

These days, it's ingrained into our minds that we can snack away to our heart's content. Hungry? Why wait? You really should reconsider this thinking. I mean if you really think about it, the current mentality of eating 6 small meals a day and snacking all the time is absurd. Think about what it was like back in the day when our parents and grandparents really frowned upon snacking before we ate our meals.

Avoid Eating For The Sake of Eating

The problem most people face is when they start embarking on a healthy lifestyle is a lower appetite. Your body actually responds with a decline in appetite. But most folks don't listen to their body and they eat and snack just for the sake of it.

I'm not against snacking. If you are hungry, please eat. Don't deprive yourself of nutrition. If you are not hungry, don't eat. Listen to your body – it's your best guide.

Breakfast is not necessarily the most important meal of the day

Once again, we are all different and there are some breakfast people and some non-breakfast people. I'm a big breakfast but that's me. How about you?

When you listen to your body's cues, there is no need to stuff yourself with food in the morning if you are not hungry. I'm letting you off the hook. However If you find skipping breakfast makes you eat like it's going out of style later in the day, then having something in the morning will work for you. If you are okay with nothing to eat until later and still keep your eating under control, then you are good to go.

Breakfast is really no more important than lunch or dinner and there is no scientific evidence that says any different. In fact, you will not find legitimate scientific studies that prove having three or more meals a day is better than one or two.

Are you asking me to starve myself?

Not at all. Let's be clear: short and flexible fasting is not about starving yourself. You are really not starving. Most people don't really know what starving is. Starvation is the images you see in the news from third world countries. Willingly skipping a meal here and there is not the same thing. Stop the melodrama.

The important question to ask is whether you are really afraid of starving yourself or if you're mentally and emotionally attached to food. Maybe you are afraid this will be difficult or painful for you as a result.

Dispelling The Misinformation and Myths About Fasting

There are a lot of people who hear of fasting and get really scared because of all the misinformation about it, so let's dispel some of the myths about fasting and metabolism.

Your metabolism is not affected by fasting

It's important to know what metabolism is. Stripping it of all the fancy science, it's basically the rate at which your body uses energy to maintain itself.

The bottom line is that food is unimportant when it comes to your metabolism. Your metabolism is affected by two common things:
1. Your weight affects your metabolism – More precisely, your lean body mass which is everything in your body that is not fat.

2. Amount of activity affects your metabolism – When there is move-
    ment in the body and you are expending energy, there will be an
    increase in metabolic rate.

Your Metabolism Will Do Just Fine While Fasting

There was a study conducted at the University of Nottingham in England
where researchers took 29 healthy people, 12 men and 17 women and
made them fast for 72 hours. They studied the effect of fasting at 12
hours, 36 hours and 72 hours. They basically found their metabolic rate
unchanged after 72 hours of fasting - 3 days without food. In fact, interest-
ingly enough, they found that their metabolic rate significantly increased
after 36 hours of fasting.

Study after study has been done to show that snacking or eating frequently
does not give you a metabolic advantage. So snack if you are really hungry,
but not because you think you are doing yourself a favor and speeding up
your metabolism.

You Will Not Lose Muscle Mass By Fasting

Another popular myth is that while you are fasting you will lose your muscle
mass – this is completely false.

Dr Alfred Goldberg and his colleagues at Harvard University made what is
probably the most significant discovery when it comes to muscle growth.
They found that if a muscle is stimulated to grow, it will grow. Full stop, end
of story. Get this - it will grow despite a lack of food, rest, growth hormone,
and anything else you can throw into the mix.

All you have to do to stimulate your muscles to grow, is to be involved
in some sort of exercise routine. As long as you are using your muscles,
they will not waste away when you are fasting. Your diet has nothing to
do with it.

Blood Sugar Levels Will Not Get Wacky And Out of control

I want to preface this by saying that you always want to check with your doctor before implementing any changes to your diet and exercise routine because this course was created for those who don't have a previous medical condition such as diabetes, so please check with your doctor.

That being said, you have probably heard dozens of times that the reason you should eat frequent meals is to keep your blood sugar levels relatively stable. The idea is that you want to eat frequently so you don't become hypoglycemic, which might make you irritable, lightheaded, and shaky.

Hypoglycemia is having abnormally low blood sugar, and it's not to be confused with hyperglycemia, which is having abnormally high blood sugar.

Hypoglycemia or having low blood sugar actually affects very few people and in fact research shows than unless you are being treated with a drug for diabetes, it's not common in healthy individuals.

The reason most people are not affected by hypoglycemia is that your body has to maintain blood sugar in a narrow range and it is remarkably efficient at regulating your blood sugar.

Over a 24 hour period, normal blood glucose levels will vary. They will increase after meals, but should drop to a lower normal level when your food has been consumed. Then overnight or during a fast there is actually only a slight reduction in blood sugar levels.

A study done at the University Hospital of Stockholm in Sweden looked at two groups of healthy adults: those who did not report hypoglycemia and individuals who said that they might suffer from hypoglycemia because they became irritable and shaky when they were not eating frequently.

What they found is that after a blood test after a 24-hour fast, no hypoglycemia was evident in either group. Individuals who said they suffered from hypoglycemia reported significantly higher scores on 'irritation' and 'shakiness' even though there was no difference in blood sugar.

The conclusion is that these symptoms were caused by the stress and anxiety over not eating and not due to low blood sugar.

Benefits of Fasting
Lose weight by burning more body fat

When you are in the fasted state, there is an increase in two important processes: lipolysis and fat oxidation. Lipolysis is the breakdown of stored fat and fat oxidation is the process of burning fat.

What this means is that fasting gives your body a chance to stop storing fat and start burning it.

There are numerous studies that point to an increase anywhere from 50 to 100% in both breaking down of fat and burning it for fuel in folks who were involved in short and flexible fasting.

Think about that – you double the amount of fat your burn in such a short period of fasting. Where do you sign up?

Creating Hormonal Harmony

The reason most diets don't work is because they fail to address the underlying root cause of weight gain, which is hormonal dysfunction. Hormones are the chemical messengers that give direction to all your bodily functions, including how much you should eat, how fit, or how fat you become. They can work for you or against you depending on what you do.

To really understand how your hormones work, we have to baseline the body and realize that when it comes to food, your body can be in only one of two states. You are either in the:
1. Fasted state, or the
2. Fed state

What hormones are present and what they do is like night and day depending on whether you are in fasted or fed state. A lot of hormonal magic happens when your body is in the fasted state.

The hormonal harmony that is created by fasting is twofold:
1. An increase in all the right hormones needed for energy and fat burning, and a
2. Decrease in insulin and an increase in insulin sensitivity.

Let's quickly examine each one of these and why they're important.

Increase in all the right hormones needed for energy & fat burning Increase in Glucagon – If insulin is the fat storing hormone that is made by the pancreas, then glucagon is the *fat burning hormone* also made in the pancreas.

Insulin takes blood sugar and converts into glycogen and then takes the excess sugar and stores it as body fat. Glucagon has the exact opposite effect. It releases glucose from glycogen and also increases lipolysis which is the release of fatty acids from stored body fat. Glucagon is only present when you are in the fasted state.

Increase in Growth Hormone – This hormone is like the elixir of youth. Growth hormone is produced by the pituitary gland in the brain and it tells your body to quickly repair itself, grow muscle, and increase the breakdown of body fat and the burning of fat.

Other natural ways to increase growth hormone include deep sleep and exercise.

The most common artificial way is to artificially inject it into the body. This is what many in Hollywood do to look younger and what some athletes do in an attempt to enhance their athletic performance. But it's not without scary side effects.

Fasting is the easiest and most natural way to increase growth hormone by up to nearly 500%. Think about that, your body is indeed the perfect pharmacy. If you give it a chance, it will create all the right hormones in the right dosage and deliver it in abundance to the target places without side effects. As a result, you look years younger, have a lot of energy, and become a fat burning machine.

Decrease in insulin and increase in insulin sensitivity

Food consumed will cause a rise in insulin and if your level of insulin is chronically high, you will store body fat and stop the breakdown of stored body fat from happening.

Short and flexible fasting has a remarkable effect on reducing your levels of insulin and insulin sensitivity so your body cells become more sensitive to insulin. As a result, you don't have to secrete as much insulin and insulin levels return to lower normal levels while you continue burning fat.

Longer Life Span and Higher Quality of Life

A few years back, I was totally fascinated by a British fellow called Buster Martin. He refused to take a day off on his birthday from his work as a van cleaner for a plumbing company. Doesn't sound terribly exciting until I actually found out that it wasn't just any birthday, it was his 100th birthday. On his 102nd birthday, he entered the London Marathon and walked the entire 26.2 miles in approximately 10 hours.

Buster Martin got me very fascinated with longevity research and what easy things people can do to increase not only their lifespan, but also their quality of life. As it is right now, human beings have the ability to live to 120 years, but right now the average life span in the United States is about 78 years old.

However, growing in our midst are the Buster Martins of the world. Those guys and gals who are 100 years old or more and scattered all over the world. They don't appear to follow a particular diet or healthy lifestyle. Some centenarians smoked. There is a woman who lived to be 122 years who had smoked most of her life. Some did not exercise regularly, some were particularly careful with their diet, others ate whatever they wanted. Actor and comedian George Burns smoked and drank his way to 100.

Now the easiest thing to say is that they hit the genetic lottery, but if you look closer, you find that it's not true. Centenarians who have a high quality of life share the following metabolic profile:

- Low fasting leptin levels
- Low fasting Insulin levels
- Lower body temperate
- Low percentage of body fat
- Reduced thyroids
- Low triglycerides (a type of fat found in your blood)

Here is the kicker: all these bio markers are improved by fasting.

Emotional Freedom From Eating Mindlessly

You will have a huge sense of emotional freedom when you adopt short and flexible fasting. In his book, "Mindless Eating," Brian Wansik, a well-known food behavior and psychology professor, says that the typical person makes about 200 decisions a day when it comes to food.

For example, if you were having breakfast, you would have to decide when to eat, what cereal to have, the bowl, what kind of milk, how much, would you want fruit, where you want to eat it, whether you want another one, when you were done, and other decisions. You've probably made a dozen decisions before you even eat it.

Remember, you don't have an infinite amount of brain resources so the more you spend fretting about food, the less you have for other important things. Many who have adopted short and flexible fasting report having a sense of freedom in their normal day because they don't have the emotional stress that comes with making all the decisions you need to make about food. Many folks report being more alert, increasing creativity, and improved memory.

It becomes emotionally refreshing when you mentally unburden yourself from the constant stress and worry about food.

How To Put into Practice Short and Flexible Fasting

1. **Allow about 12 hours between your last meal and first meal of the day – Every day of the week**
   Sleep and early morning are prime fat burning times. All the hormones needed for burning fat, such as glucagon and growth hormone, are at high levels. Most folks go 6 – 8 hours without eating in the morning. All I'm asking you is to try to increase that to around 11 or 12. For some, this is not difficult for others it might take a little work. If you find that 8 hours is as much as you can do, add an hour or two until you are able to get to 12. This might take a couple of weeks or a few months so be patient with yourself.

2. **Eat Real Meals and Limit Snacking**

   Listen to your body when it comes to food and don't force yourself to snack. Don't eat for the sake of eating and please don't mistake this for an all or nothing deal. Please eat or snack if you are hungry because your activity level will vary from day to day, it's your call to make, but if you aren't hungry, don't eat. Listen to your body. Most days I eat 2 times per day. When I'm very active it could be 3 or more. If you are honest with yourself, you will know when you are eating just for the sake of it.

3. **Fast once or twice a week for 20 – 24 hours**

   Here is where you give yourself the wonderful gift of a digestive vacation. Take a break from eating once or twice a week for 20 – 24 hours. This is easy because you never go for a day without eating.

   This is how the magic happens. 2 -4 hours after your last meal, depending on the size of your meal, your body begins breaking down fat and burning it. The amount of fat burned is steadily increased until about the 12th hour and at this point most of what you are burning is mostly body fat. Another jump also happens around the 18 hour mark until the 24 hour mark where there is an increase in about 50% in fat burning.

How To Implement Your Weekly Fast

Short and flexible weekly fasting is exactly that, it's short and flexible. It's flexible because there are no exact times, or days for you to begin and end your fast, you can fit it into your personal lifestyle.

For example, if you have dinner at 7:00pm, then 24 hours would be 7:00pm the next day and 20 hours would be subtracting 4 hours from 7:00pm which is 3:00pm the next day.

Importance Of Timing

Timing is very important because it will determine your success. You will find that fasting during certain times of the day to be tough. If you find the beginning of the fast is too tough, then begin your fast in the evening. For example, begin your fast at 6:00pm so you are able to go to bed and are asleep when the fasting becomes too tough for you.

Many people will find the middle or the end of the fast tough, so my suggestion is try fasting late morning around say 11:00am or my personal favorite around 1:00pm. It's not really a one-size-fits all, but the flexibility allows for you to work it around your specific needs.

Nothing is set in stone, so if there is a surprise party that comes up on your fasting day, simply move it to the next day or another time during the week. No harm, no foul.

People like to say that you never get something for nothing but by using short and flexible fasting you are basically getting great results by doing absolutely nothing.

There are three stages you need to be aware of to be successful with your fast.
1. Preparation
2. The actual fast
3. Breaking the fast

Each one of these stages is important so let's take a look at them.

Preparation:

You have to be prepared both physically and mentally.

Mental Preparation

Mental preparation begins with knowing when you are going on your 24-hour fast. I recommend having a set day of the week for this. When you get really good after doing these for say 3 months or more, you could do it on the fly so you decide that perhaps today or tomorrow would be a good day to fast but when you are starting out, I highly recommend that you plan the day of fasting in advance.

The more you plan something, the better you will be at following through. Things happen, life changes, but when you plan it's the best way to mentally prepare for your fast – or for anything in your life. As Eisenhower once said, "Plans are worthless, but planning is everything."

Make your chosen fast day a firm decision because if you set your mind in advance then you will not start deliberating during your fast whether you should continue or not. The moment you start questioning yourself, you will always find a gazillion reasons why you should start eating.

If you have this kind of determination and set your intention beforehand, then your desire to eat will greatly diminish when you start fasting. What happens is that your appetite for food almost shuts down. This always amazes me but you have to experience this for yourself.

Physical Preparation Before You Fast

Don't overeat. Eat as your normally do prior to fasting. Don't overeat and think you can make up for not eating during your fast. This is very bad idea because it backfires on you. Before your fast, eat as your normally would.

Stay Hydrated – Remember, it's important to be properly hydrated before starting your fast. Drink filtered water or filtered alkaline or drinking lots of wheat grass is the best thing for you to do.

During fasting, drink a lot of water to make sure you are properly hydrated. Most of the time when you believe you're hungry - you are actually just thirsty. The reason for this confusion is that the signals for both hunger and thirst are very similar and we very easily mistake thirst for hunger. In addition the effects of dehydration such as tiredness and persistent hunger are often experienced the following day so before you fast make sure you are properly hydrated.

During The Fast

During your fast, once again make sure you are properly hydrated. Since your body is not trying to deal with digestion it will start to expel and eliminate toxins en masse. Help the process of flushing the debris by drinking water. You may also drink zero calorie beverages such as black, green or herbal teas, black coffee, and sparkling water.

The only thing I want you to be particular about is to keep your calories on your drinks to zero as much as possible. The moment you start adding cream and sugar, it can negatively affect the effectiveness of your fast. The only exception that I make is that you can drink your wheat grass during this time, because even though it has very few calories, it's very alkalizing and is packed with a lot of nutrition with a negligible effect on your digestive system.

Diet sodas are okay even though I like to discourage drinking of diet sodas because the caffeine, carbonation, and all the other junk they have in most diet sodas will increase the acidity of your stomach which means you naturally want to eat something to calm the acid.

The one thing you don't want to drink is any sort of juice natural, fresh squeezed, or otherwise because this totally negates the reason for fasting which is having close to zero calories as possible.

Stay busy

Have you ever heard the phrase that an idle hand's are the devil's workshop? There is some truth because you will find it easier to fast when you are busy and mentally stimulated.

When you lack mental stimulation, you are more likely to use food and snacking as stimulation. Don't plan to sit at home and watch movies while fasting because you are making it harder on yourself. Try to stay busy.

Breaking The Fast

When your fast is done, you should be very proud of what you have accomplished, but try your best to treat it like a non-event. It's normal in the beginning of practicing short and flexible fasting that you might over eat. Remember it's a process and you will get better at it, don't be too hard on yourself just try better next time. Don't make it an occasion that requires over indulgence of a special food treat, reward, or celebration. In other words, just eat the way you normally would.

Can You Exercise While Fasting?

The answer is a resounding YES. The benefits of exercising are enormous and they will only speed up your weight loss results. Whatever fitness program you have and more importantly, enjoy doing is fine. I encourage both cardio and resistance training as you can do both while fasting and enjoy even better results.

Exercise can help you burn a lot of fat while fasting, but key is figuring out if you are training for results or performance. What I mean is do you want to burn fat or are you trying to meet a certain goal like beating a certain time or running a specific distance.

I don't recommend exercising while fasting for endurance events like marathons or triathlons or for improving physical performance such as beating your time in running or cycling events. If physical performance is your goal, then find a different day other than your competition days.

However, for the vast majority, you can still be in the middle of 24 hour fast and workout while fasting. Not only will you have a wonderful workout, but you get to burn a lot more fat than you ever have.

Mistakes to avoid while doing Short and Flexible Fasting
Avoid Over Enthusiasm

This is when you are told to take two pills by the doctor and you decide because you want to get better you take the whole bottle. It's important to take it slow.

Don't try to fit in as many fasts in the week. Once or twice is what I recommend otherwise you will experience fasting burn out.

Don't extend your fasts beyond the 24 hours either. Yes, you will experience quick results, but you will also experience "fasting burn out". Enjoy your life, enjoy the joys of eating but take it slow.

If you start fasting for more than once or twice a week and for longer than 24 hours, you might start dreading your next fast and that's not what you want or need. You want this to become a lifestyle, one that you really enjoy especially after you start witnessing the results you get.

Stop Being Hard On Yourself

If you are relaxed and flexible, you will have a much better experience and even better results. Instituting short and flexible fasting is not meant to cause stress in your life. If you are on your 20-24 hour fast and you get to the 18th hour and you find yourself eating, it's okay. You did not fail. Don't beat yourself up.

Remember what I said about thinking of progress and not perfection?

If you find yourself not sticking to your plan, ask yourself questions like possibly starting at a different time of day. If you succumbed to a specific food was it a craving or because you were in close proximity to it? Was it stress? Ask questions without judging yourself and try to figure out if you are able to do better next week. So next week try for 19 hours. Don't obsess about it, just allow yourself to experience what happens when you take a break from eating and just try to do better every time.

Module 4: Summary

We talked about the following short-term fasting techniques:
1.   On a daily basis allow a minimum of 11 or 12 hours between your last meal and first meal of the day.
2.   Don't snack or eat if you are not hungry, eat real meals instead.
3.   Fast once or twice a week for 20 – 24 hours.

At a bare minimum I want you to try the fasting once or twice a week for 20 – 24 hours, but for extraordinary results, do all three.

Remember don't be hard on yourself if you fall short. If on your 24-hour fast you don't quite get to 20 or 24, don't sweat it, you will still benefit. I want you to learn from your experiences and remember you don't have to be perfect.

MODULE 5

Taming Appetite, Behavior, and Cravings

The ABC's of Weight Loss

Appetite, behavior, and cravings - I call these three the ABC's of weight loss. If you are able to have a good handle on these three things, you will lose weight. And you won't have to use willpower.

The reason this is an important module is because it deals with hunger. I don't need to tell you this, hunger is a powerful force. When we get hungry, nothing else seems to matter. It's hard to fight hunger because it's a genetic response because it almost always wins.

The reason you easily lose your temper when hungry is because of an increase in your adrenaline levels. Nature wanted our primitive ancestors, regardless of hunger, to go into the jungle without fear and hunt and kill for food.

Real hunger is primal and a lot more severe. It's the pictures from the 6 o'clock news you have seen of people starving from third world and developing countries. Real hunger is not just an empty stomach. Real hunger is not knowing where your next meal will come from.

Habits Are Everything

Our eating habits determine everything. There is quote from Jim Rohn that I love: "Motivation is what gets you started but habit is what keeps you going." Now there are two reasons for our eating habits. One is physiological - your body's needs tell you when and how often you should eat. The other is psychological - your mind and emotions make that bulk of decisions often independent of what your body's needs are.

Getting Your Mind and Body In Sync

It's really important to get both your mind and body in sync when it comes to your cravings and appetite. The goal is to still enjoy your food and feel satisfied without dramatic changes in your diet. Food is more than just a physical thing. It's also emotional as well and a very powerful force in our lives. Marilyn Migliore, author of the book, "The Hunger Within," says it so well, "Food is the number one mood-altering substance we all use."

The Love and Food Connection

We made the link between food and comfort as babies. We were held in nurturing arms and as we were constantly fed, we knew food was love. When we cried, we were fed. As kids, when we did something good, we celebrated with food, like ice cream. For example, I was with my nieces at the hospital because they were not feeling well and they were given lollipops for a brave visit at the doctor's office.

We celebrate birthdays with cake, Christmas with cookies, Thanksgiving with turkey, and a milestone achievement such as a promotion with a fancy dinner. Food is a backdrop for so many of our favorite activities, like watching a movie or a sporting event.

Our emotional link for food is deep in our subconscious too. If we don't like how we feel, we eat; if we like how we feel, we eat. We seem to gain weight when things are going so well, or when life seems to be falling apart at the seams. Food is an emotional thing that's not just limited to a few people, it's in all of us.

At one point or another, we have all engaged in emotional eating and truth is that we will continue to do so. The important distinction to make is how often you do it and also if you are even aware you are doing it.

Emotional eating is not about feeding your body, it's about feeding your emotions and this happens every time you eat for reasons other than hunger.

You know That You Are Eating Emotionally When

1. You suddenly feel hungry. Physical hunger is a gradual process that happens over a period of time.
2. You crave and immediately want to eat a specific type of food. You feel that only this particular food will satisfy your appetite. Physical hunger is happy to get what it can, while emotional hunger is focused on specific tastes and textures.
3. You eat unconsciously, so suddenly you're eating ice cream and you find the whole container is gone.
4. You continue to eat, despite being satisfied or overly full.
5. You are left with feelings of guilt after pigging out.

Mental Tools For Handing Emotional Eating

Here are two important tools for handling emotional eating:
1. Awareness without guilt or shame
2. Self talk

Awareness Without Guilt or Shame

First, let me say that you are allowed to eat emotionally. Yes, emotional eating is part of being a human being. What gets you in trouble is using it exclusively to handle the ups and downs of life and overdoing it. Like with most things in life, too much of something is not good.

When you catch yourself eating emotionally and beating yourself up over it, try to stop both. If you can't stop eating immediately, that's okay because you will get full and stop at some point. The most important thing is that you don't beat yourself over it, just enjoy what you're eating without guilt or shame.

Guilt is feeling you have done something wrong while shame is feeling that we ourselves are bad for something we have done. These are very tricky emotions that cause us so much unnecessary suffering.

Release feeling guilty over all your shortcomings in life – it's not worth it. Feeling guilty or ashamed over something you have done does not make you a better person instead it's punishing yourself. This sort of self-abuse does not prevent you from repeating your mistakes. Instead, it's the beginning of a vicious cycle. In the end guilt/shame often drive you to repeat the same thing over and over again.

Has this ever happened to you? You decide that you are on a diet and exercise program. But the first day you slip and miss a workout and perhaps binge on some cake, you feel guilty. And what do you do? You feel so guilty that you punish yourself by having more cake or ice cream. Then you feel even more guilt and pretty soon the diet is a distant memory.

Instead, the solution is to learn being a witness or an observer of your life. The truth is your actions are brought about by your thoughts and feelings which just don't come out of nowhere. So become a witness to your thoughts and actions, **without judging** yourself because the moment you start being critical of what you are doing, the witnessing stops, you become involved and you miss a lot of important information.

How to increase awareness and be a witness to your life

All you have to do is watch your thoughts and actions without guilt or judgment by noticing what you are doing and just say to yourself "that's interesting"

From this place, you can only clearly review the mental tape of your thoughts and actions by observing with curiosity. You want to be curious about your feelings and actions without being critical. If you are just curious, you will be amazed at what have been missing when it comes to emotional eating.

All emotional eating stimuli comes from our five senses – sight, taste, smell, touch, or hearing. Watch with curiosity the origin of the thoughts you have and how you behave. You will begin to find out the most fascinating things about your cravings and appetite. You'll learn how colors and certain sounds, even music, can make you crave certain foods.

Awareness without being critical of yourself is enough to make you change.

You become an observer of your own life as you witness all the internal and external processes that happen for you to create your unhealthy habits. You can become this independent, non-critical and non-judgmental observer of all you do just by saying to yourself the two words "that's interesting".

This is how you observe with curiosity and bear witness to your life, and doing this without criticizing yourself is enough to make you change.

Because once you witness yourself do something that does not serve you, you will soon find yourself unable to keep repeating it.

Self Talk

Talking to ourselves is something each one of us does. We could no more stop talking to ourselves than we could stop breathing. All we can do is to try to control the nature and the direction of those internal conversations we have.

Most people are totally unaware that our inner conversations control the direction of our lives and how we act and behave are a result of these inner conversations.

The one thing you must do is to choose your words carefully when you want to lose weight. Make no mistake about it, the words you use are as powerful as sticks and stones.

I recall an interesting study that pointed out that people who were in the habit of saying the word 'sick' with passion like "He or she makes me sick" would often fall sick days later. There are many religious texts that say that the world was created just with words. Make no mistake about it, the words we use are how we often we create the circumstances in our lives.

There are two words that we need to avoid using if you want to control your internal conversation when it comes to food.

Love

Love is the word we commonly throw around when it comes to food. Do you love pizza, chocolate or pasta? Really? Do you love these foods like you love your kids or family? Or if you believe in a high power or higher intelligence, do you love these foods more than your creator or your closest of friends? Of course not. But these errors in language and little lies that we tell ourselves affect us and radically change our eating habits.

Don't say you LOVE eating pizza or chocolate or whatever you like to eat, instead say you ENJOY it and your mind and body will begin to respond differently to it.

As human beings we have very strong associations for the word love. Leave it for when it really counts and avoid having food in the love category because you can get in trouble.

Starving

"I'm starving" or its cousins like "famished", "I could eat a horse" and "dying of hunger". You get the point. Are you REALLY starving? Do you really know what starving is? Starving are those people from developing countries that are close to their death beds on the news. Could you really eat a horse? REALLY?

Check your language and be careful of what you say, because your subconscious mind can make some very powerful associations with food.

Why? Because when it comes time to eat and after continuously telling yourself all these little lies about your state of hunger, your body will not know that they were just words. And what ends up happening is that you get into the horrible habit of eating more than you need because subconsciously your body thinks that you might not eat again for a while.

How To Help Your Body Control Appetite and Cravings

There are two parts to controlling your appetite, behavior, and cravings. One is mind, which we just covered, and the other is body. These are things you can physically do to make it easier for you to control all three critical areas: appetite, behavior, and cravings when it comes to weight loss.

See Food Diet!

Have you heard of the joke about the person who claims to be on the 'see food diet'? This is because whenever they see food, they eat it. It's funny but true. A study was published in the late 60's by Dr Stanley Schachter which showed that obese individuals tend to eat according to external factors or triggers that seem to originate outside of the stomach. The sight of food was the biggest one. Others include smell, time of day, advertisements and strong emotions such as stress or sadness.

The truth is that everyone is on the 'see food diet'. We like to eat what we see. Research expert Brian Wansik shows that if you take the candy dish that many office workers like to place on their desk and move it about 6 feet away, it will make you eat close to 60% less candy and result in about 12 less pounds of weight you have to battle during the year.

Apply this to your home and make getting access to tempting foods inconvenient.

Shrink Your Stomach

When you begin to eat less, you actually begin to shrink your stomach, which is a muscle by the way. It is a muscle that can expand and contract, depending on how much food you constantly eat. It's a simple equation: smaller stomach, smaller appetite, more fullness, and fewer cravings.

The first thing you must know about eating is that you are not supposed to continue eating until you are stuffed. You are supposed to eat until you feel you are not hungry anymore. This is a very important distinction to make.

Three Stomach Settings

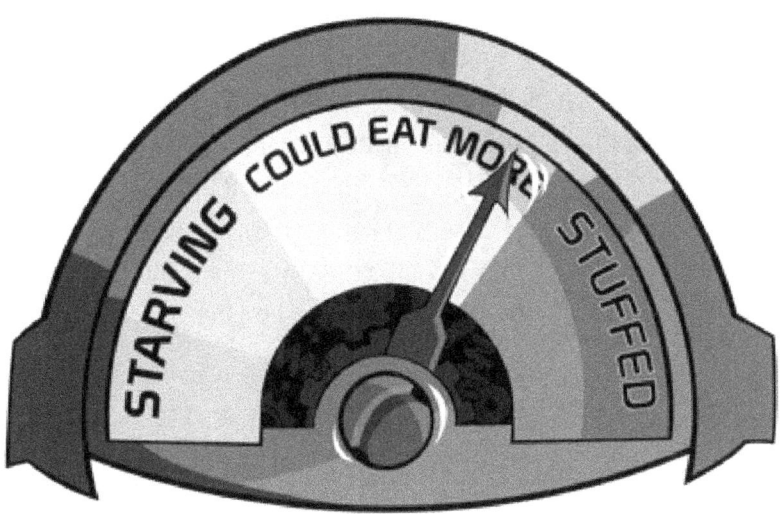

The stomach seems to have three settings:
1. Starving
2. Could eat more and
3. Stuffed.

The goal is to learn the skill of listening to your body when deciding when you are not hungry anymore. There is a difference between too little and too much food and an area in the middle where you are not hungry but not stuffed either. This is where during a meal, you know you could always eat more, but instead it's where you should choose to stop.

This is easier said than done so here are the three things you can physically do to control your appetite, behavior, and cravings

Some of these will look familiar.

Control Cravings and Appetite By Eating More Fat, Especially Good Fat

Eating good fats will make you less hungry between meals and have fewer cravings. Having more of the good fats especially your daily tablespoons of oil will help increase feelings of fullness which means you will eat less during meals and not want to snack between meals. It has also shown to prevent your insulin levels from spiking when you do consume sugary foods. Eating more good fats will also greatly reduce the headaches you get when you eat less carbs, especially when you fast.

Control Cravings and Appetite By Eating More Fiber

The act of adding fruits to your breakfast and veggies, nuts and beans to your lunch will give you that feeling of early satisfaction in a meal without adding too many calories. This action makes you feel full faster and for much longer which means you are less likely to be hungry a couple of hours after eating.

Control Cravings and Appetite By Chewing More – Get Sugar Free Chewing Gum

What really makes us full has baffled scientists for a while but it seems to be combination of how much food we visually see, taste and for how long we've been chewing. Chewing seems to be the biggest contributor to satiety. This third tip is enough to dramatically reduce your appetite and will be a breakthrough for a lot of you.

The foods we consume today have become less crunchy/chewy because of processing and modern science. We did a lot more chewing back in the day when most of what we had were nuts, fruits, and vegetables. Foods these days are cooked, processed and very convenient.

Back in the day, even when we ate meat it was not a burger. It was meat that required a fair amount of chewing. Eating was not a 10 minute affair like it is these days; it took an hour.

Enter your most powerful weapon – sugar free gum.

But you need to use sugar free gum correctly to see the best results.

1) Chew gum 15 – 30 minutes before you eat

The right way to reduce your hunger, cravings, and appetite is to chew gum 15 to 30 minutes before you eat.

Drink water before or while you are chewing gum for the best results. When it comes time to eat, it will literally feel like you have been eating for the last 30 minutes or so and you will feel full faster.

2) Chew gum after your meal

Remember you are not supposed to eat until you are full, but we all know it's hard to stop. Eat until you are not hungry then pop in a piece of sugar free gum, chew and sip on some water. This is my favorite technique for not over eating.

The signal that travels between your stomach and your brain that tells you that you are full is on a 15 to 20 minute delay. Chewing gum will give you something to do that feels like eating while giving this signal enough time to be received by brain.

Chewing sugar free gum while properly hydrated will significantly reduce your cravings. You will eat less food and not feel deprived. This also has a snowball effect because the less you eat the smaller your stomach becomes and the less food you need to make you feel full.

What are the best chewing gums?

Most sugar free gums contain 1 to 3 calories; so having some while doing your short and flexible fasting is fine. I have found that chewing gum during short and flexible fasts is also very helpful - just don't forget to drink water while doing so.

What gum should you buy? There are many chewing gums out there that are all natural, using xylitol instead of artificial sweeteners. I've tried many of these organic and natural gums but I personally find they are not as easy to chew and long lasting as one of my favorite brands that has a little artificial sweetener but I think it's worth the exemption because of the goodness it does for you.

The sugar free gum I prefer to chew is made by Wrigley's and is called 5 (Five). The flavor I like is called cobalt, but find something you like.

Module 5: Summary

Learn to be an independent and judgment free observer of your life and actions and watch yourself with curiosity as you respond to emotional eating cues. Don't beat yourself up when you catch yourself eating emotionally, instead be curious about your thoughts and feelings by saying to yourself, "that's interesting." Once you see yourself create an outcome that does not serve you, you will soon find yourself unable to keep doing it.

Be careful with the words you use when it comes to food and appetite association. Avoid using the word LOVE for food because the truth is that you really don't LOVE eating a particular kind of food. You might enjoy eating it, but that is not love. Use LOVE for people and other things that really matter to you.

Other words to avoid using are STARVING or 'eating a horse' or other exaggerations. These little lies get into your subconscious and you find yourself pigging out because you keep telling yourself that you are starving and your body responds by overeating.

One thing you can physically do to control your appetite, behavior, and cravings is to eat more good fat. I recommend daily tablespoons of healthy oil, eating more fiber, and chew some sugar free gum 15 to 30 minutes before your meal and immediately after your meal while sipping water.

FINAL THOUGHTS

Let's answer a burning question most people have:

What Exactly Should I Eat?

You will not find me filling this course with recipes because that is not the point. The goal is for you to adopt this quick and easy way of losing a lot of body fat with your current lifestyle. Eat the foods you like but use the guidelines I've provided. My recommendation is simple: enjoy eating better food less often.

There is room for a good, delicious meal, even a dessert. What gets us in trouble is how often and how much we indulge. I'm 100% confident that with my program you will still enjoy your favorite foods while losing weight and getting healthy.

When it comes to food, I like to encourage you to eat real food and less processed foods. The goal is to get foods that are as close to their natural state as possible. This means eating the orange and not drinking orange juice. This also means, if you are going to have meat, having real meat and not the processed stuff like hot dogs, bologna, and other packaged meats.

The picture below is the end product of mechanically separated chicken.

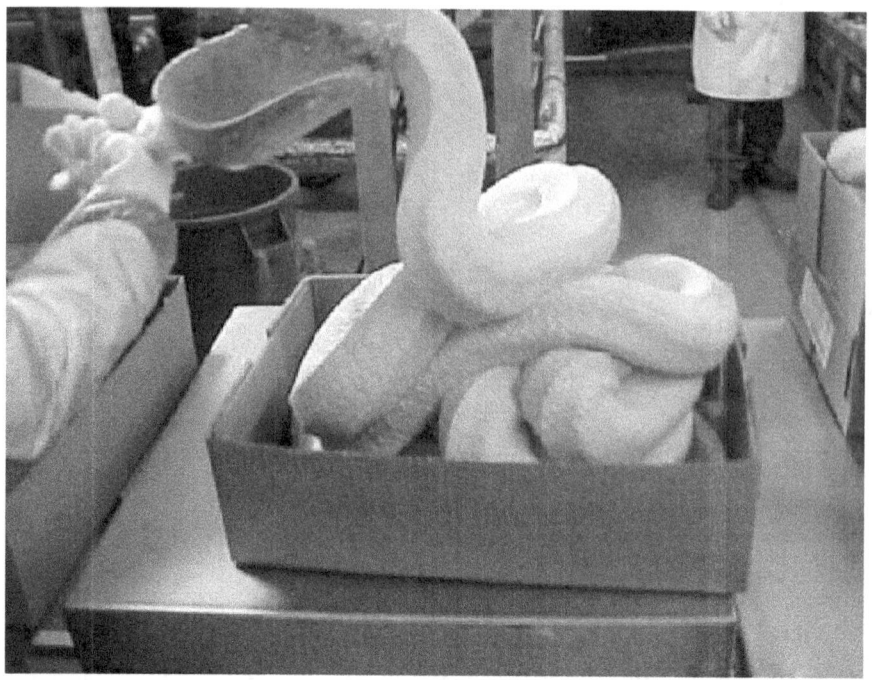

Yes, this pink gunk looking substance is the stuff they use to make chicken nuggets and other processed meats like hot dogs and bologna. It's the result of a process called **Advanced Meat Recovery (AMR)**. This is what meat producers do to increase their profits. They use the last traces of usable meat from bones and all the parts of an animal such as intestines, eyeballs, and tendons and grind it all out into a paste that looks pink.

Then, because it's crawling with bacteria, they soak it in ammonia and because there is really no taste, they artificially add flavor to it. The final step is to add artificial coloring to it to make it look edible because no one wants to eat a pink chicken nugget.

"Real Food" Guidelines

Eating doesn't have to be so complicated and author Michael Pollan of the book "Food Rules," lays out a set of straightforward simple guidelines that I like. Here are a few of the simple things that resonate with me:

- If it came from a plant, eat it, If it came from a factory, avoid it.
- Avoid eating anything your great grandmother wouldn't recognize as food. So when you pick up something with 15 ingredients, most of which you can't pronounce, ask yourself, "What are those things doing there?"
- Avoid food that won't eventually rot. Things like Twinkies that never go bad aren't real food.
- Avoid buying food where you buy your gasoline. In the U.S., 20% of food is eaten in the car.

Avoid Eating Foods With Artificial Ingredients and Chemicals

Karen Hanrahan, a wellness educator and nutritional consultant, has kept a McDonald's hamburger since 1996. Her point was to show that unlike a normal hamburger, McDonald's hamburgers don't decay. Look at the picture below. Can you guess which one is 12 years old?

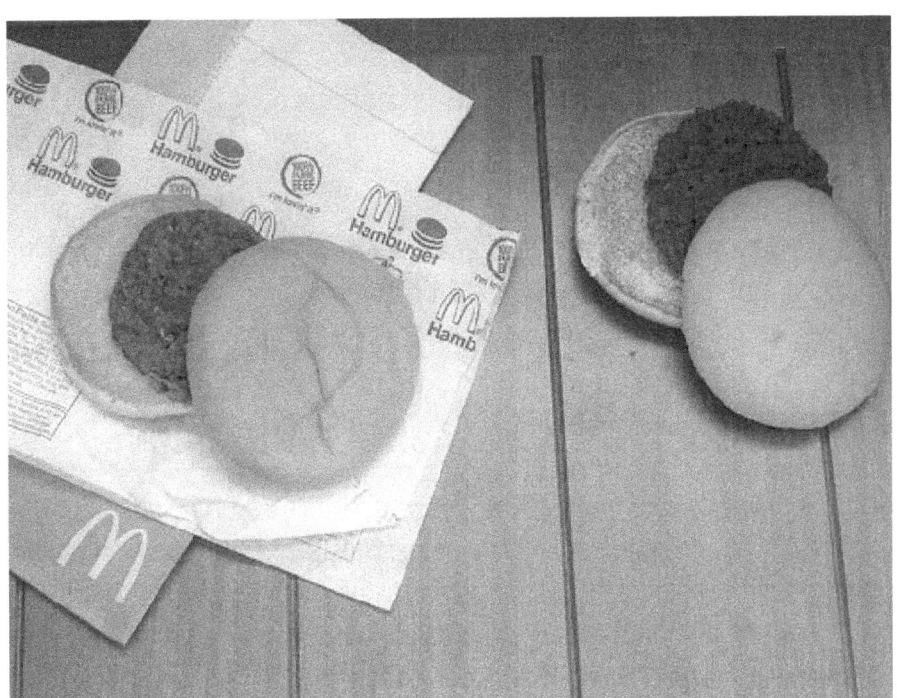

The brand new McDonald's hamburger is on the right and the one on the left is from 1996 and both look edible.

Processed foods contain a lot of chemicals designed to preserve the food, enhance flavor, bulk it up, etc. Even if they are low in calories, the chemicals in the food are treated as a poison that the body has to eliminate, and this job falls on the liver.

Remember the liver does hundreds of functions in the body. For example it produces substances that break down fats and it also helps maintain the proper level of blood sugar by storing glucose as glycogen. The amazing liver also makes certain amino acids that are the building blocks of proteins, and also stores minerals and vitamins such as vitamins A, D, K and B12. The liver is the body's largest internal organ and out of the hundreds of roles it performs, the filtering of harmful chemicals from the blood takes top priority.

So when you eat processed foods that have all those chemicals that the body cannot absorb, the job falls on the liver to remove them. These chemicals are treated as a poison and detoxification takes precedence over everything else. Your liver now has to stop doing all the other things it supposed to do like helping you burn fat, because its busy filtering out all the chemicals you have dumped in it.

Has this happened to you? You are doing your work and your boss comes to your office and shouts about an emergency problem that needs your full attention. Do you think you will do the other stuff that you were working on before? Probably not.

Making Comfort Food More Comforting

Don't deprive yourself but become a food detective and read your labels – avoid eating foods that contain the word 'artificial' in their list of ingredients. If you are going to indulge, get quality stuff. Keep your comfort foods but eat them in small amounts because a small amount will take you a long way. My goal is to get you eating better, but less often.

The Beginning...

This will indeed be a new beginning for you and the countless number of people you will impact with a healthier more energetic body. I also want to say thank you for buying this course because life is more fulfilling when we can pay it forward. I hope you can gently educate those you love on how they too can sleep fat and wake up thin.

I also want to offer my heartfelt congratulations. Very few people follow through on their commitments and if you have gotten to this point you already possess what is needed for you to make all the required changes in your life.

Now with all this information you have, turn it into real knowledge by using it and customizing into your life. You might not implement all ideas at the same time but those you start doing right now will make a tremendous difference. This is life changing stuff and I cannot wait for you to write to me and tell me about your success stories.

This book is about nutrition and as a result we did not talk about exercise but it's important. Drum roll please because I'm going to reveal the secret of getting excellent results with exercise. Are you ready? It's **consistency.**

Remember Buster Martin from Module 1? 102 years old, in excellent shape and for exercise all he does are push ups every day!

My friend, it's really that simple. Find some enjoyable exercise or daily movement you like to do and do it everyday.

My danceX workout is my pride and joy. It's fun, easy to follow has great music and delivers fantastic results. One of my promo videos on YouTube has over 1.9 Million hits!! and people from all around the world have bought my DVDs to learn more about it, go now to my website http://www.danceX-fitness.com

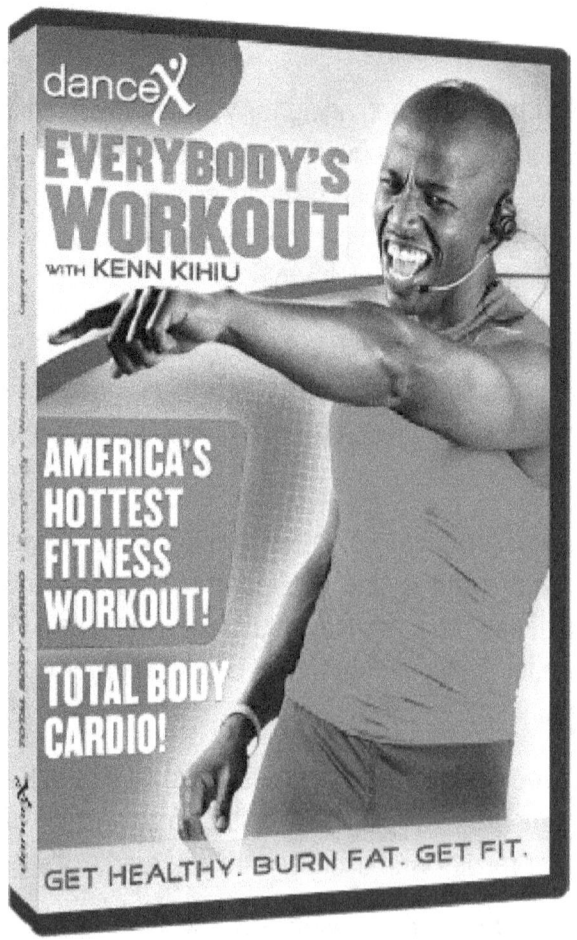

Above is a picture of my danceX workout DVD. To learn more visit my web-site http://www.danceXfitness.com

Questions Or Comments

I'd love to hear from you, tell me about your results or your thoughts. You can email me at **kenn@dancexfitness.com**

You have all my love and I wish for you the best life has to offer. Here is to the beginning of your abundant health, happiness, and success.

Health, Happiness & Success

Kenn Kihiu

P.S

Special Thanks

Gratitude is a driving force in my and from the bottom of my heart I want to thank all my clients and customers worldwide wherever you are.

Thank you for being a part of my life, you inspire me, encourage me to do more, create more and be more. You make me a better human being.

I love my work — my life's mission and the only reason I can do this is because of you. Everyday I whisper a silent heartfelt thank you.

P.P.S

One Last Thing...

In this day and age there are plenty of ways to easily reach and influence those you care about. I would like to invite you to rate this book and *share your thoughts through Facebook and Twitter.* If you think your friends and family will get something valuable out of this book, I'd be honored if you'd post your thoughts.

If you feel particularly strong about the contributions this book will make to achieving your goals, I'd be eternally grateful if you posted a <u>review on Amazon</u>.